RAND NATIONAL DEFENSE RESEARCH INSTITUTE

T0127933

Complementary and Alternative Medicine in the Military Health System

Patricia M. Herman, Melony E. Sorbero, Ann C. Sims-Columbia

Prepared for the Office of the Secretary of Defense

For more information on this publication, visit www.rand.org/t/RR1380

Library of Congress Cataloging-in-Publication Data
ISBN: 978-0-8330-9511-4

Published by the RAND Corporation, Santa Monica, Calif.

© Copyright 2017 RAND Corporation

RAND® is a registered trademark.

Support RAND
Make a tax-deductible charitable contribution at
www.rand.org/giving/contribute

www.rand.org

Preface

Complementary and alternative medicine (CAM) is made up of a variety of therapies (e.g., acupuncture and chiropractic) that developed outside the conventional biomedical model of care. CAM is used by about one-third of the general population and offered within the military health system (MHS). However, no systemwide data are available on its use.

In order to improve patient care by assuring the safety, quality, and consistency of these services through informed policy decisions, the Defense Center of Excellence for Psychological Health and Traumatic Brain Injury (DCoE) asked RAND to conduct an environmental scan/survey of CAM services in the MHS to understand the extent to which CAM and integrative medicine (IM) practices are available in military treatment facilities (MTFs), the types of available services, the conditions for which these services are used, and the types of providers who deliver these services and their privileges and credentials. This report presents the results of this survey, which was fielded in 142 MTFs across the three branches of service (Army, Air Force, and Navy) and the National Capital Region Medical Directorate (e.g., Walter Reed).

This research was sponsored by DCoE and conducted within the Forces and Resources Policy Center of the RAND National Defense Research Institute, a federally funded research and development center sponsored by the Office of the Secretary of Defense, the Joint Staff, the Unified Combatant Commands, the Navy, the Marine Corps, the defense agencies, and the defense Intelligence Community. For more information on the RAND Forces and Resources Policy Center, see www.rand.org/nsrd/ndri/centers/frp.html or contact the director (contact information is provided on the web page).

Contents

Preface iii

Figures vii

Tables viii

Summary ix

Acknowledgments xvii

CHAPTER ONE

Background 1

What is CAM? 1

How Widely Is CAM Used? 2

Conditions for Which CAM Is Used 3

Purpose of This Report 3

CHAPTER TWO

Methodology 5

The CAM Survey 5

Use of CAM Services in MHS Utilization Data 7

Strengths and Limitations of Our Study 8

CHAPTER THREE

CAM Prevalence Across MTFs 11

Types of CAM Services Offered 14

What Evidence Do MTFs Use When Deciding to Offer CAM Services? 16

CAM Use as Reported in the MHS Utilization Data 18

To What CAM Services Do Conventional Providers Refer Patients? 20

Prevalence of CAM: Key Points 21

CHAPTER FOUR

Conditions and Diagnoses for Which CAM Is Used 23

How Is CAM Being Used? 23

Do Patients Adhere to Treatment, and Is It Effective? 24

Use of CAM in MTFs—Key Points 26

CHAPTER FIVE

Demand for CAM Services at MTFs 29

How Often Do Patients Request CAM? 29

How Often Are CAM Services Used?.. 30
Comparing Estimated Patient Encounters and Actual Patient Visits................................. 34
Are Patients Waiting for CAM Services?.. 35
Demand for CAM: Key Points... 36

CHAPTER SIX
Practitioners Who Provide CAM at MTFs 37
Who Delivers CAM, and How Much Time Do They Spend? 37
CAM Clinical Settings and Integration of CAM into MTFs... 38
How Much Is Invested in CAM Annually? 40
Who Is Responsible for Credentialing and Privileging CAM Providers? 42
Training of New CAM Providers.. 43
Practitioners Who Provide CAM at MTFs: Key Points.. 44

CHAPTER SEVEN
CAM Coding and Documentation...45
CAM Coding and Documentation: Key Points 48

CHAPTER EIGHT
Summary and Recommendations 49

APPENDIXES
A. Acupuncture at a Glance..53
B. Chiropractic at a Glance...57
C. Diet Therapy at a Glance 61
D. Mindfulness Meditation at a Glance... 65
E. Stress Management/Relaxation Therapy at a Glance... 69

Appendixes F–H are available at
    http://www.rand.org/pubs/research_reports/RR1380.html

Abbreviations.. 73
References 75

Figures and Tables

Figures

S.1.	Number of CAM Services Provided in MTFs ($N = 133$)	x
S.2.	Conditions for Which CAM Use Is Most Commonly Reported by MTFs and CAM Services Most Commonly Used for Each	xii
S.3.	Patient Encounters per Month in MTFs for Most Commonly Offered CAM Services ($N = 110$)	xiii
1.1.	Types of CAM by Commonly Used Groupings	2
3.1.	Reasons MTFs Do Not Offer CAM Services ($N = 18$)	11
3.2.	Reasons MTFs Offer or Plan to Offer CAM Services ($N = 115$)	12
3.3.	Number of CAM Services Provided in MTFs ($N = 133$)	13
3.4.	Type of Evidence Used to Support the Decision to Provide CAM Services for the Ten Most Commonly Offered CAM Services	19
3.5.	Frequency of CAM Use 2008 to 2013 by Type of CAM, MHS Utilization Data	20
3.6.	CAM Services Reported as Among Three Most Commonly Referred to by Conventional Health Care Providers at MTFs Offering CAM ($N = 110$ MTFs)	21
4.1.	Conditions for Which CAM Use Is Most Commonly Reported by MTFs and CAM Services Most Commonly Used for Each	23
4.2.	Types of Diagnoses for Which Outpatient CAM Was Used in 2013, MHS Utilization Data	24
4.3.	Reported Levels of Perceived Patient Adherence for CAM Services Most Frequently Offered by MTFs	25
4.4.	Most Common Benefits from CAM Services per Patient and Provider Report and the CAM Services Most Often Reported as Showing That Benefit	27
4.5.	Reported Reduction in Medication Use Among Users of CAM Services	27
5.1.	Frequency of Providers' Receipt of Requests from Patients for CAM Services ($N = 133$)	29
5.2.	Patient Encounters per Month in MTFs for Most Commonly Offered CAM Services ($N = 110$)	30
5.3.	Five CAM Services Offered in MTFs with the Most and Least Patient Encounters per Month	33
5.4.	Estimated Frequency of Patient Encounters per Month Across All MTFs, by Specific CAM Services	33
5.5.	Number of Patients on a Wait List at MTFs for Commonly Offered CAM Services	36
6.1.	Number of FTEs Accounted for by MTF Staff and Contractors/Volunteers of Different Provider Types, All CAM Services Provided in MTFs	38

6.2.   Clinical Settings in Which CAM Services Are Offered in MTFs ($N = 110$) 40
6.3.   Estimates of MHS Labor Investment in CAM by CAM Type and Provider Type 41
6.4.   Entities Responsible for Reviewing and Approving Clinical Privileges for
       Providers Delivering the CAM Services Most Commonly Offered at MTFs 42
6.5.   Types of Training Given to CAM Providers When They Start Working in
       MTFs ($N = 110$) 43
7.1.   MTFs That Reported Consistent Documentation of Common CAM Services
       in the EMR 45
7.2.   CPT Procedure Codes Used to Document Common CAM Services in MTFs 46
A.1.   Acupuncture Procedures in 2013 MHS Utilization Data 54
B.1.   Chiropractic Procedures in 2013 MHS Utilization Data 58

Tables

S.1.   CAM Services Provided at MTFs, CAM Survey Data ($N = 110$ MTFs) xi
2.1.   Current Procedural Terminology (CPT) and International Classification of
       Diseases, Ninth Revision (ICD-9) Procedure Codes Specific to CAM Therapies 7
2.2.   Clinical Classifications Software Groups Used In this Report 8
3.1.   Number of CAM Services Provided in MTFs by Branch of Service 13
3.2.   Number of CAM Services Provided in MTFs by MTF Size 14
3.3.   CAM Services Provided at MTFs, CAM Survey Data ($N = 110$ MTFs) 15
3.4.   How CAM Services Are Offered and Reported at MTFs, CAM Survey Data 17
4.1.   Number of Outpatient CAM Services Used for Each Type of Diagnosis in 2013,
       MHS Utilization Data 25
5.1.   CAM Service Combinations that MTFs Reported as Having >500 Patient
       Encounters per Month 31
5.2.   Patient Procedures and Visits from MHS Utilization Data Compared with
       Estimated Patient Encounters from CAM Survey 34
6.1.   Numbers of Outpatient CAM Procedures Delivered by Different Types of
       Providers in MTFs, by Type of CAM in 2013 MHS Utilization Data 39
7.1.   CAM Activities Captured in CPT Codes 47

Summary

Complementary and alternative medicine (CAM) comprises a large number of therapies that developed outside the conventional biomedical model of care. Fairly well-known examples of such therapies include acupuncture and chiropractic care. CAM is used by about one-third of the general population—including services administered by a CAM provider (e.g., acupuncture) and therapies that can be practiced outside of a health care setting and/or are self-administered (e.g., yoga). Its use has been found to be higher in some populations—including active-duty military members and those with particular conditions, such as posttraumatic stress disorder (PTSD).

CAM is known to be offered within the military health system (MHS). However, this report provides the first systemwide look at the CAM services offered in the MHS. The Defense Centers of Excellence for Psychological Health and Traumatic Brain Injury (DCoE) asked RAND to conduct this environmental scan and data collection effort in order to obtain initial data on the availability, documentation, coding, credentialing and privileging practices, and demand for CAM services across all military treatment facilities (MTFs). These data on current CAM practices will be used to inform policy decisions on the use of CAM in the MHS, on credentialing and privileging of those who provide CAM, and on documentation of its use to support ongoing monitoring and assure safety, quality, and consistency of these services.

Methods

This study consisted of two components: the development, fielding, and analysis of data from a survey of CAM services offered in MTFs; and a supplemental analysis of MHS health care utilization data to assess the frequency of CAM procedures offered across the system.

The CAM Survey

The CAM survey was adapted from the 2011 Veterans Health Administration (VHA) CAM Survey, which was used to capture information about CAM services in the VHA in 2011.

The study was designed to be a census of MTFs. The Assistant Secretary of Defense for Health Affairs tasked the Assistant Secretaries of Manpower and Reserve Affairs in each military service to circulate the data call to all the MTFs under their purview, which resulted in the identification of a total of 142 MTFs. The survey was completed during August through October 2015. Overall, responses were submitted for 133 of 142 MTFs, resulting in a response rate of 94 percent.

MHS Utilization Data

In a complementary effort, we assessed CAM utilization using MHS health care utilization data for all active-component service members across outpatient and inpatient health care provided at and outside the MTFs. Our analyses focused on CAM practices for which procedure codes exist: acupuncture, biofeedback, chiropractic, hypnosis, and massage. We examined trends in CAM utilization for fiscal years 2008 through 2013. Additional analyses focused on the 2013 data to increase comparability to the results of the survey.

Results

Prevalence of CAM

According to the survey, most MTFs (83 percent) offer CAM services, usually from one to eight different types (Figure S.1). The number of CAM services offered differs substantially across service branches. Army MTFs offer a larger number of CAM services; the Air Force is the least likely to offer CAM. MTF size also is associated with CAM offerings: Larger MTFs are both more likely to offer CAM and a wider range of services.

The most common types of CAM that MTFs offer are stress management/relaxation therapy, acupuncture, progressive muscle relaxation, guided imagery, chiropractic, and mindfulness meditation (Table S.1). MTFs reported offering CAM services individually and as a package with other CAM services (e.g., relaxation therapy and progressive muscle relaxation). Acupuncture and chiropractic are the two CAM services that MTFs are most interested in offering whether or not they offer them currently. The majority of MTFs reported using scientific evidence and experiential or anecdotal evidence in their decision to offer specific CAM services. The main reasons MTFs offer CAM are (1) as an adjunctive to chronic disease management (80 percent); (2) to fulfill patient preference (74 percent); (3) to promote wellness

Figure S.1
Number of CAM Services Provided in MTFs (*N* = 133)

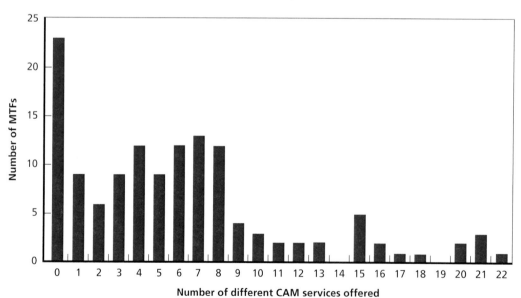

Table S.1
CAM Services Provided at MTFs, CAM Survey Data (*N* = 110 MTFs)

CAM Service	*N*	Percentage
Stress management, relaxation therapy	83	75
Acupuncture	76	69
Progressive muscle relaxation	64	58
Guided imagery	61	55
Chiropractic	60	55
Mindfulness meditation	56	51
Diet—special, diet therapy	52	47
Dietary/nutritional supplements	43	39
Biofeedback	39	35
Acupressure	30	27
Yoga	29	26
Other meditation	26	24
Massage therapy	22	20
Movement practices	16	15
Animal-assisted therapy	15	14
Hypnosis/hypnotherapy	15	14
Music therapy	15	14
Tai chi, qi gong	11	10
Dry needling	11	10
Osteopathic manipulative therapy	11	10
Aromatherapy	10	9
Mantram repetition meditation	10	9
Energy healing	9	8
Nontraditional spiritual practice	8	7
Traditional Chinese medicine	8	7
Other	7	6
Transcendental meditation	6	5
Herbal medicines	6	5
Hyperbaric oxygen therapy	6	5
Chelation therapy	0	0
Ayurveda	0	0
Homeopathy	0	0
Native American healing practices	0	0
Naturopathic medicine	0	0

(72 percent); and (4) because of proven clinical effectiveness (66 percent). Half of MTFs report that they offer CAM because it promotes cost savings. Lack of provider availability and a lack of provider awareness and interest are the primary reported reasons why MTFs without CAM services do not offer them. A lack of patient interest in CAM and MTF worries about safety or efficacy were rarely reported as barriers to offering CAM.

Chiropractic services occurred with the highest frequency in the 2013 MHS utilization data, followed by massage, and acupuncture. Thus, while the CAM survey indicates more MTFs offer acupuncture than chiropractic, more patients are receiving chiropractic care.

Conditions for Which CAM Is Used

Across MTFs, CAM is most often used for chronic pain, stress management, anxiety, back pain, and sleep disturbance (Figure S.2). Acupuncture and combinations of mind-body medicine therapies were in the five CAM services most often reported as being used to treat each of those conditions. Acupressure and chiropractic were included in the five CAM services most commonly used for the two pain conditions (chronic pain and back pain), and progressive muscle relaxation and stress management/relaxation therapy were in the five most commonly used for the three psychological health conditions (stress management, anxiety, and sleep disturbance).

MTFs reported CAM services were most effective at improving quality of life, reducing pain, reducing stress, reducing anxiety, and improving patient satisfaction. Acupuncture, mind-body medicine combinations, and stress management/relaxation therapy were all in the five CAM services most often associated with all these improvements. Chiropractic was one of the five most commonly associated with improved quality of life, reduced pain, and improved patient satisfaction, and mindfulness meditation was one of the five most often associated with reduced stress and anxiety. More than half of the MTFs that reported acupuncture and chiropractic as showing success in the treatment of pain, depression, anxiety, PTSD, or sleep disturbance also reported they were associated with reduced medication use.

Figure S.2
Conditions for Which CAM Use Is Most Commonly Reported by MTFs and CAM Services Most Commonly Used for Each

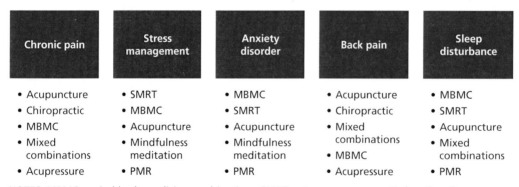

Chronic pain	Stress management	Anxiety disorder	Back pain	Sleep disturbance
• Acupuncture	• SMRT	• MBMC	• Acupuncture	• MBMC
• Chiropractic	• MBMC	• SMRT	• Chiropractic	• SMRT
• MBMC	• Acupuncture	• Acupuncture	• Mixed combinations	• Acupuncture
• Mixed combinations	• Mindfulness meditation	• Mindfulness meditation	• MBMC	• Mixed combinations
• Acupressure	• PMR	• PMR	• Acupressure	• PMR

NOTES: MBMC = mind-body medicine combinations; SMRT = stress management/relaxation therapy; PMR = progressive muscle relaxation.

Reported patient adherence tended to be higher for manipulative and body-based therapies (e.g., acupuncture, acupressure, chiropractic, and massage) than for mind-body interventions (e.g., meditation, progressive muscle relaxation [PMR]) or biologically based interventions. This could be because patients often have to practice the latter two on their own.

Patient Demand for CAM

Forty percent of MTFs reported that their providers received frequent requests for CAM services. Half of the MTFs that do not offer CAM services report that patients rarely requested CAM, while 13 percent report frequent requests for CAM services. This could reflect a lack of interest in CAM at MTFs not offering these services or simply awareness that they were not available in the MTF.

There is substantial variation—both across type of CAM and across MTFs—in the monthly number of patient encounters in which these CAM services are used alone (Figure S.3). Approximately two-thirds of MTFs reported fewer than 50 patient encounters per month for five of the ten most commonly offered CAM services: acupuncture, stress management/relaxation therapy, progressive muscle relaxation, biofeedback, and acupressure. Patient volume is much higher for chiropractic: Only 10 percent of MTFs reported fewer than 50 patient encounters per month, and almost 20 percent reported more than 500 chiropractic patient encounters per month. Based on information provided by MTFs, the total estimated number of patient encounters was almost 76,000 (45,500 to 106,000) per month. Estimates were generally consistent with observed frequencies in MHS utilization data for CAM practices with procedure codes.

Wait lists are one measure of unmet demand. Wait lists for most commonly offered CAM services are uncommon and short when they do exist. However, approximately 45 percent of

Figure S.3
Patient Encounters per Month in MTFs for Most Commonly Offered CAM Services (N = 110)

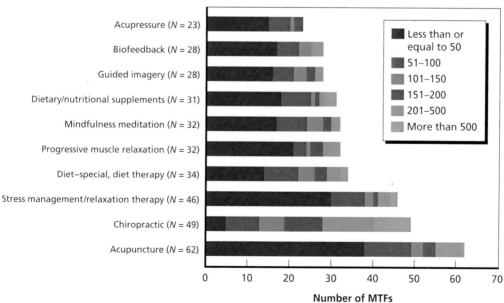

MTFs reported a wait list for chiropractic and acupuncture with one-third to one-half of the wait lists consisting of more than 40 people.

CAM Provider Types, Clinical Setting, and Their Credentialing and Privileging

Physicians (MDs/DOs), clinical psychologists, and licensed social workers provide more than half of the total 1,555 full-time equivalents (FTEs) of MTF staff time devoted to CAM, based on MTF estimates. Based on this FTE estimate and estimates of the average annual salary for each category of provider, the total MHS labor investment in CAM in 2015 is approximately $112.7 million. Of this, the majority ($100.8 million) is MTF staff (versus contractor) time.

MTFs report that most CAM services are offered in outpatient settings, consistent with what was seen in the MHS utilization data. The majority of MTFs reported that CAM services are offered in primary care, followed closely by outpatient behavioral health and outpatient pain clinics. About one-third of MTFs report that they deliver at least some of their CAM services in an integrative health/medicine clinic, or a CAM specialty clinic. The most common sources of CAM referrals are primary care, followed closely by referrals from psychologists, psychiatrists, or other behavioral health providers, and self-referral or referral from friends or family.

Credentialing and privileging is a process to ensure qualified providers deliver health care. At least 80 percent of MTFs report having a credentialing board or committee or other form of review process for most of the commonly offered forms of CAM. However, 30 percent of MTFs report not having an established process for mindfulness meditation.

Coding and Documentation

More than half of MTFs report that commonly offered CAM services are "consistently documented in the electronic medical record (EMR), Armed Forces Health Longitudinal Technology Application (AHLTA)," with at least 90 percent of MTFs reporting consistently documenting chiropractic and acupuncture. However, up to one-third of MTFs were uncertain about the consistency of documentation for many common CAM services. In addition, documentation is not as consistent for less-commonly-offered CAM services.

At least 60 percent of MTFs reported that no Current Procedural Terminology(CPT) codes exist for six of the ten most commonly offered CAM services (stress management/relaxation therapy, acupressure, dietary and nutritional supplements, mindfulness medication, guided imagery, progressive muscle relaxation). When MTFs reported using CPT codes for these CAM services, the codes used suggested that some MTFs use related CPT codes or generic visit codes even when specific CPT codes exist for a CAM service (e.g., acupuncture or chiropractic).

Conclusions and Recommendations

This report provides the first systemwide look at the CAM services offered in the MHS. It also highlights substantial variation across MTFs in the types of CAM offered, frequency of use when services are offered, coding practices, and the privileging and credentialing of providers offering CAM. Our two sources of data each have limitations. Individuals assigned to this task at each MTF collected the CAM survey data. Respondents reported that they obtained the requested information by talking to individual CAM providers, staff in behavioral and mental health and in primary care, and other health care providers. In MTFs that offer just a small number of CAM services, it is likely that a single individual or small group of people have adequate knowledge to accurately answer the survey. However, larger MTFs with numerous clinics may provide CAM services of which the MTF respondent was unaware, or a small group of people may not have sufficiently comprehensive knowledge of the CAM services provided to accurately answer all the questions in the CAM survey. We are grateful for their efforts but hope that this report will highlight the need for more formal and consistent systemwide data collection.

The health care utilization data that we used to supplement the CAM survey also has limitations. Specific procedure codes are available for only five general types of CAM: acupuncture, biofeedback, chiropractic, hypnosis/hypnotherapy, and massage therapy. Therefore, analyses based on the MHS data could address only those five therapies. The CAM survey results suggested some confusion in the availability of codes, and how best to record the provision of CAM services in utilization data, which would affect estimates of CAM use. First, multiple MTFs reported a lack of CPT codes for CAM such as acupuncture when such codes do exist, which would lead to an underestimate of CAM services used. For CAM for which codes to not exist, some MTFs reported using related codes (e.g., using acupuncture codes for the provision of acupressure), which would lead to an overestimate of some CAM services, or the use of generic visit codes, which would lead to the use of CAM services not being identified in our analyses. The net effect of these conflicting inconsistencies is unknown.

However, despite the limitations in our data sources, our systemwide assessment of CAM services in the MHS makes an important contribution to ongoing efforts to understand the role of CAM in this context in order to better inform policies related to its provision and use. To further the goal of understanding the role of CAM in the MHS, we offer the following recommendations:

- **Standardize coding for CAM services.** More systematic data collection will allow for consistent tracking of the types of CAM services being offered, their provider types, and the conditions for which they are used, will allow better manpower management, a better record for physicians about the other treatments that patients are receiving, and easier data collection for future comparison studies.
    - Standardized coding should be developed for CAM services for which no specific CPT code currently exists.
    - Because a number of CAM services are offered in combination (by the same provider for the same conditions and often in the same session), a standard way of coding should be developed for a predefined set of these combinations.
- **Conduct a medical record review at a small number of MTFs to validate survey findings and MHS utilization data.** MTFs report that almost all CAM use is consistently documented in the EMR, so these records could be used to validate the data collected through the CAM survey—particularly the types of CAM offered, conditions for which CAM is used, the providers who are delivering these therapies and the time devoted to the provision, and patient encounters per month. Furthermore, given the reported incon-

sistency in the use of procedure codes to record CAM, a medical record review could also validate MHS utilization data for CAM in the selected MTFs and could guide the standardization of CAM coding.

- **Address CAM in clinical guidelines for conditions for which it is frequently used.** More than half, but not all, of MTFs cited scientific evidence as a reason to offer their CAM therapies. Addressing CAM in the clinical guidelines will facilitate providers having access to the scientific evidence on the safety, efficacy, and effectiveness of CAM therapies for specific conditions and should help support better-informed decisions by MTF commanders, clinical leaders, and individual providers about the types of CAM to offer and conditions these therapies are best used to treat in all MTFs. DCoE has initiated this process by funding a series of systematic reviews for selected CAM services and conditions, which have informed Department of Veterans Affairs (VA) and Department of Defense (DoD) clinical guidelines. We encourage the continuation of this activity prioritizing the high-frequency condition–CAM combinations identified in this report.
- **Standardize credentialing and privileging.** A standardized protocol for credentialing and privileging the providers of CAM services should be developed to ensure that the providers are properly and consistently trained, and to assist MTFs in credentialing and privileging new CAM providers.
- **Target future research toward the CAM services with reported success.** Future research might appropriately target condition–CAM service combinations associated with reports of symptom improvement and/or medication reduction, especially if other MTFs want to offer them, and/or sufficient relevant clinical studies do not already exist.

Implementation of these recommendations may have important implications for patient care by assuring the safety, quality, consistency, and appropriate availability of CAM services.

Acknowledgments

We gratefully acknowledge our project officers and points of contact at the Defense Centers of Excellence for Psychological Health and Traumatic Brain Injury—Mark Bates, Brad Belsher, Chris Crowe, Justin Curry, Michael Freed, Marina Khusid, Katherine McGraw, and Angela Steele—for their support of our work. We also acknowledge the support of our points of contact for each of the service branches: Richard Niemtzow and Rene Chadwell (Air Force); Joseph Phillips and Kevin Galloway (Army); Moira McGuire (National Capital Region Medical Directorate); and Fredora Green-McRae and Joan McLeod (Navy). We appreciate the comments provided by our reviewers, David M. Benedek and Carrie Farmer. We addressed their constructive critiques, as part of RAND's rigorous quality assurance process, to improve the quality of this report. We acknowledge the support and assistance of Alerk Amin, Dionne Barnes-Proby, JoEllen Fielden, Gina Frost, Ujwal Kharel, Jeremy Kurz, Darryl Metcalf, Sherry Oehler, Marc PunKay, Teague Ruder, Timothy Smith, Mary Vaiana, Christine Vaughan, and Kayla Williams in the development of the data collection instrument, fielding of the data collection effort, analysis of the data, and preparation of this report. We are grateful to Kristie Gore for her support and guidance throughout the project. Finally, last but not least, we are grateful for the time and effort of the military treatment facility staff who gathered and submitted data on their MTFs and made this study possible.

CHAPTER ONE

Background

Complementary and alternative medicine (CAM) comprises a range of therapies that developed outside the conventional biomedical model of care. Fairly well-known examples of CAM therapies are acupuncture and chiropractic care. Historically, CAM therapies were not offered within the conventional or mainstream health care system. However, their use by the public is pervasive (Clarke et al., 2015), and they are gaining attention as options for pain and psychological health beyond opioids and other medications (Menard et al., 2014). CAM is currently used in the military health system (MHS) (Goertz et al., 2013; Jacobson et al., 2009; Smith et al., 2007; White et al., 2011); however, there is no systemwide data on the types of CAM services offered or the frequency of their use.

This study provides the first comprehensive picture of the availability of CAM across the MHS and the conditions for which CAM is used. We also report on patient demand for CAM, provider credentialing and privileging, referrals and collaboration between CAM and conventional practitioners, and perceived effectiveness of the therapies. Sound credentialing and privileging are essential to maintaining the quality of any kind of health service, and they would ensure that the practitioners who provide CAM services are properly trained. In addition, perceived effectiveness helps identify CAM therapy and condition candidates for future outcomes research. We also explored the documentation and coding of CAM services in MHS utilization data. Good documentation of CAM use is necessary for ongoing monitoring of the expansion of CAM and how it is used over time and will help to ensure the safety, quality, and consistency of its utilization, as well as facilitate better tracking of manpower use and needs.

What is CAM?

The term *complementary and alternative medicine* is in a state of flux. For years, the National Center for Complementary and Alternative Medicine (NCCAM), a component of the National Institutes of Health (NIH), defined CAM as "a group of diverse medical and health care systems, practices, and products that are not generally considered part of conventional medicine" (National Center for Complementary Alternative Medicine, 2012). Although this definition in essence still stands today, the term CAM has been more recently replaced by other terms, mainly variations on complementary and integrative medicine or health. As an example of this change, NCCAM is now called the National Center for Complementary and Integrative Health (NCCIH), and the NCCIH website now refers to "health care approaches developed outside of mainstream Western, or conventional, medicine" (NCCIH, 2015a). NCCIH's website goes on to describe integrative medicine: "There are many definitions of 'integrative' health care, but all involve bringing conventional and complementary approaches together in a coordinated way" (NCCIH, 2015a). Despite the recent flux in terminology, this report will use the term CAM. Most CAM use occurs in conjunction with conventional medicine (Institute of Medicine Committee on the Use of Complementary Alternative Medicine by the American Public, 2005; NCCIH, 2015a).

While the range of CAM therapies is quite extensive, CAM services are typically broken into five general categories (see Figure 1.1) (Healthcare Analysis & Information Group, 2011; Institute of Medicine Committee on the Use of Complementary and Alternative Medicine by the American Public, 2005; NCCIH, 2015a). Each type of CAM is described in the glossary (Appendix G).

How Widely Is CAM Used?

Approximately one-third of adults in the United States ages 18 and older report using some form of complementary health approach in the past 12 months—a statistic that has been fairly constant for more than a decade (Clarke et al., 2015). CAM is used for a wide variety of physical and psychological conditions, and most often as an adjunct to conventional medicine (Institute of Medicine Committee on the Use of Complementary Alternative Medicine by the American Public, 2005; NCCIH, 2015a). CAM also is used for general improvement of health and well-being (Barnes, Bloom, and Nahin, 2008; NCCIH, 2015b).

Current CAM use in the U.S. military is slightly higher than the rate of use seen in the U.S. population as a whole, with recent estimates of the prevalence of past-year CAM use in active-duty military populations ranging from 37 percent to 45 percent (Goertz et al., 2013; Smith et al., 2007; White et al., 2011). Two surveys of active-duty personnel in smaller clinic settings reported somewhat higher CAM use—49 percent and 72 percent (Kent and Oh, 2010; McPherson and Schwenka, 2004), but this higher use in these clinic-based samples may be in part because CAM users reported more illness and poorer health in general (Jacobson et al., 2009; Smith et al., 2007; White et al., 2011).

Figure 1.1
Types of CAM by Commonly Used Groupings

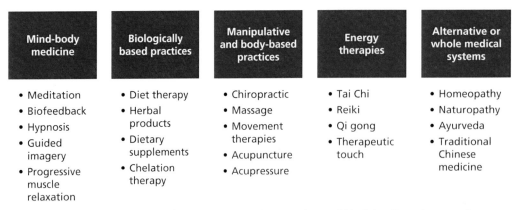

SOURCES: Healthcare Analysis & Information Group, 2011; Institute of Medicine Committee on the Use of Complementary and Alternative Medicine by the American Public, 2005; NCCIH, 2015a.
RAND RR1380-1.1

Some types of CAM are more commonly used in military populations. Chiropractic care was integrated into military health care in the 1990s (Lott, 1996). Currently, chiropractic, acupuncture, clinical nutrition therapy, meditation, yoga, and massage therapy are some of the most commonly reported types of CAM services offered (Department of Defense [DoD], 2014); these therapies plus guided imagery, relaxation therapy, herbs, and high-dose megavitamins and minerals are some of the most common types of CAM used by military personnel (Goertz et al., 2013; Smith et al., 2007).

Over time, CAM service offerings at military treatment facilities (MTFs) have increased. Interviews with the Deputy Chief of Clinical Services or service equivalent in 14 selected MTFs in 2005 and 2009 revealed a substantial increase in the number of providers delivering CAM, number of MTFs offering different types of CAM, and the types of CAM services offered (Petri Jr. and Delgado, 2015). A 2014 report to Congress indicates that 29 percent (120) of 421 MTF departments reported offering a total of 275 CAM programs in calendar year 2012 (DoD, 2014).

Conditions for Which CAM Is Used

CAM is utilized for a wide variety of physical and psychological conditions, as well as for general improvement of health and well-being (Barnes, Bloom, and Nahin, 2008; NCCIH, 2015b). A national sample of the U.S. population indicates that the 15 most common conditions for which CAM is used are back pain, neck pain, joint pain, arthritis, anxiety, cholesterol, head or chest cold, other musculoskeletal, severe headache or migraine, insomnia or trouble sleeping, stress, stomach or intestinal illness, depression, and regular headaches (Barnes, Bloom, and Nahin, 2008). The one study available that indicates the conditions for which CAM is used in a military population generally replicates this list (McPherson and Schwenka, 2004). One general population study of individuals who met the DSM-IV diagnosis criteria for PTSD indicates that 39 percent of those individuals use CAM (Libby, Pilver, and Desai, 2012).

As evidence mounts and is summarized, the use of CAM is being incorporated into clinical practice guidelines. For example, the current Department of Veterans Affairs (VA) and DoD clinical practice guidelines for posttraumatic stress disorder (PTSD) and major depressive disorder (MDD) recommend selected CAM modalities as an adjunct, or as an alternative, to front-line treatments after all have been tried and found ineffective for the patient (Management of MDD Working Group, 2009; Management of Post-Traumatic Stress Working Group, 2010). For MDD, the herb St. John's wort and light therapy are recommended. For PTSD, acupuncture and CAM therapies that facilitate a relaxation response (e.g., mindfulness, yoga, acupuncture, massage, and others) are recommended. The joint VA–DoD clinical practice guideline for the treatment of low back pain recommends several CAM therapies (spinal manipulation, acupuncture, massage therapy, yoga, and progressive muscle relaxation) as non-pharmacological therapies with proven benefits (Chou et al., 2007).

Purpose of This Report

Although CAM use in the MHS is growing, no comprehensive description of CAM offerings exists on which to base future decisions about these services in the system. To address this need, the Defense Centers of Excellence for Psychological Health and Traumatic Brain Injury (DCoE) asked RAND to conduct an environmental scan and data collection effort in order to obtain initial data on the availability, documentation and coding, credentialing and privileging practices, and demand for CAM services in each MTF. This information can be used to better inform policies regarding the future availability of CAM services across the MHS, as well as manpower use and training needs relating to the provision of CAM. In addition, the information on CAM coding and documentation could provide the basis for guidance for providers on better recording of the provision of CAM services. We also analyzed MHS utilization data (administrative data on health care utilization across the military health system) to determine the extent to which CAM services are recorded in these data and to obtain additional estimates of patient encounters and the provider types delivering CAM.

Our discussion is organized as follows:

- Chapter Two describes the methods for the CAM survey (including the development of the survey instrument and sampling procedures) and a secondary analysis of MHS utilization administrative data to identify CAM procedures used in the MHS.
- Chapters Three through Seven highlight key findings on CAM services in MTFs based on the CAM survey and, where applicable, findings from the analysis of MHS administrative data.
- Chapter Eight contains conclusions and recommendations.
- Appendixes A through E summarize the key results and characteristics for five CAM services commonly offered and used at MTFs: acupuncture, chiropractic, diet therapy, mindfulness meditation, and stress management/relaxation therapy.
- Appendixes F and G contain the CAM survey instrument and a glossary of CAM services, respectively.
- Appendix H contains detailed results tables from the CAM survey and from the MHS administrative data analyses. Individual tables in this appendix are referenced in Chapters Three through Seven.

CHAPTER TWO

Methodology

Our study has two components: development, fielding, and analysis of data from an environmental scan/survey of CAM services offered in MTFs; and a supplemental analysis of health care utilization data to assess the frequency of CAM procedures offered across the MHS. We describe the methodology for each component in this chapter. These data sources describe the extent of CAM use across the MHS. Information on the evidentiary base for the safety and efficacy or effectiveness of the CAM therapies discussed is beyond the scope of this report.

We obtained human subjects research protection approval from RAND's Human Subjects Protection Committee and the USAMRMC Human Research Protections Office for both components of this study. The CAM survey also received approval for internal DoD data collection from the Washington Headquarters Services.

The CAM Survey

Development of the CAM Online Survey

The CAM survey was adapted from the 2011 Veterans Health Administration CAM Survey, an instrument used to capture information about the provision of CAM services in the VA in 2011 (Healthcare Analysis & Information Group, 2011). In order to compare results of the CAM and VA surveys, many of the items in the CAM survey replicate the exact wording from the VA survey. Additional questions were included in the CAM survey to obtain more detailed information on the provision of CAM within the MHS. Survey topics included

- the types of CAM used at each of the MTFs
- the conditions for which each treatment is used, with a focus on psychological health and traumatic brain injury (TBI)
- perceived effectiveness of CAM for various conditions, and whether related medication reductions were observed
- the numbers and types of practitioners providing each type of CAM and the training, credentialing, and privileging of these providers
- the evidence used to decide whether to offer CAM services at the MTF
- the demand for CAM services—based on estimated number of patient encounters per month, the number of requests providers receive, and the existence and size of wait lists
- how the use of CAM services is documented and coded
- how CAM services are provided—clinics, collaboration, referrals, etc.

To ensure that the instrument was both understandable and applicable to the MHS, the survey was reviewed internally within RAND by military fellows familiar with the MHS and by researchers with expertise in military health services. The RAND team revised the instrument with each round of feedback and invited and incorporated, where relevant, comments from DCoE. For ease and accuracy in data entry, the survey was then programmed for online completion. The final version of the survey instrument and the glossary of CAM services provided to respondents are in Appendixes F and G, respectively.

Study Sample

The study was designed to be a census of MTFs and included all Air Force, Army, National Capital Region Medical Directorate (NCRMD), and Navy and Marine Corps MTFs. The Assistant Secretary of Defense for Health Affairs tasked the Assistant Secretaries of Manpower and Reserve Affairs in each service branch with circulating the data call to all the MTFs under their purview. Therefore, the Surgeons General of each service identified all their MTFs. The data call memo was sent to the identified 142 MTFs by the Surgeons General with instructions to identify a point of contact (POC) for the data collection effort. That POC was given an MTF-specific login code and link to the online survey instrument and was encouraged to gather the data needed from suggested resources (e.g., CAM providers, staff in pain clinics) at a designated MTF. The RAND team provided technical support, sent reminder emails, and responded to questions about the scan content via phone and email throughout the data collection period.

The survey was fielded August through October 2015. The response rate was high: 133[1] of 142 MTFs (94 percent) completed the survey.

Statistical Analyses

To describe CAM services offered at MTFs and characteristics of specific services, we computed univariate frequency distributions and percentages. Fewer than 5 percent of MTFs had missing data on any given survey item. The denominators are reported for percentage calculations and indicate the number of MTFs responding to a question—e.g., questions posed to all MTFs ($N = 133$), questions posed only to MTFs that offer CAM ($N = 110$), and questions posed only to MTFs offering a particular type of CAM (N's varied).

In order to minimize data entry burden, reflect the way services are delivered in practice, and support clearer answers about provider time spent delivering CAM services and credentialing processes, survey respondents were allowed to group therapies that tended to be used together by the same practitioner for the same conditions. Respondents then answered a set of CAM service-specific questions for their defined combination(s) rather than for each of the individual therapies. Where possible, we categorized these combinations according to the types of CAM services included—e.g., combinations of mind-body therapies. Unfortunately, a large number of respondents reported on unique CAM combinations that included multiple classes of CAM services (e.g., combinations of mind-body therapies and biologically based practices) and could not otherwise be categorized. In this report, this mixed combinations group is only

---

[1] A completed survey was defined as completion of the section on CAM services offered at or recommended outside the MTF (i.e., at least Part II of the survey as shown in Appendix F). One hundred and thirty MTFs went on to also provide answers for the full remainder of the survey instrument.

considered in the discussions of patient encounters and staff time where its contribution to these estimates is substantial and informative.

Use of CAM Services in MHS Utilization Data

We used MHS health care utilization data to determine the extent of CAM utilization documented in these data. The specific files used in this analysis were extracted from the MHS Data Repository, which is managed and maintained by the Defense Health Agency (DHA). The data set contains health care utilization for fiscal years 2008 through 2013 for all active military and activated guard and reserve component service members separated into files containing outpatient and inpatient health care provided at MTFs and outpatient and inpatient health care purchased outside of MTFs. We examined these data to determine how frequently CAM therapies with existing specific codes (Table 2.1) were used.

To identify the conditions for which the CAM therapies were used, we first grouped use of CAM by diagnostic categories using the Agency for Healthcare Research and Quality Clinical Classifications Software (CCS) groups. These CCS groups are each defined by a mutually exclusive underlying set of International Classification of Diseases, Ninth Revision (ICD-9) diagnosis codes. We then grouped the CCS groups into the four general diagnosis and condition groups (see Table 2.2) and used these to describe the conditions for which CAM is used.

Each of the CCS groups listed in Table 2.2 had at least one visit in 2013 (the most recent year available in our data set and the data year used for the majority of the MHS utilization data analyses in this report) coded as using one of the CAM therapies shown in Table 2.1. The CCS groups are listed within each grouping in terms of decreasing number of events—

Table 2.1
Current Procedural Terminology (CPT) and International Classification of Diseases, Ninth Revision (ICD-9) Procedure Codes Specific to CAM Therapies

CPT Codes	ICD-9-CM (Inpatient Only) Procedure Code	CAM Treatment
90880	94.32	Hypnosis/ hypnotherapy
97124		Massage
97810 97811 97813 97814	99.91 99.92	Acupuncture
90875 90876 90901 90911		Biofeedback (with or without psychotherapy)
98940 98941 98942 98943		Chiropractic manipulative therapy
	93.84	Music therapy

Table 2.2
Clinical Classifications Software Groups Used In this Report

General Diagnosis and Condition Group	CCS Groups Included
Psychological health	• [651] Anxiety disorders • [660] Alcohol-related disorders • [650] Adjustment disorders • [657] Mood disorders • [663] Screening and history of mental health and substance abuse codes • [661] Substance-related disorders • [659] Schizophrenia and other psychotic disorders
TBI and neurologic pathology	• [095] Other nervous system disorders (includes intracranial infections and nerve disorders) • [084] Headache, including migraine • [653] Delirium, dementia, and amnestic and other cognitive disorders • [233] Intracranial injury[a] • [093] Conditions associated with dizziness or vertigo • [227] Spinal cord injury
Chronic musculoskeletal pain	• [205] Spondylosis; intervertebral disc disorders; other back problems • [212] Other bone disease and musculoskeletal deformities • [254] Rehabilitation care; fitting of prostheses; and adjustment of devices • [211] Other connective tissue disease • [204] Other nontraumatic joint disorders • [232] Sprains and strains • [209] Other acquired deformities • [225] Joint disorders and dislocations; trauma related • [203] Osteoarthritis • [202] Rheumatoid arthritis and related disease • [054] Gout and other crystal arthropathies
Other conditions	• [256] Medical examination and evaluation[b] • [257] Other aftercare (mostly postsurgical care) • [259] Residual codes; unclassified[c] • All other groups (about 2 percent of CAM visits)

[a] This diagnosis group contains a number of the TBI-related ICD-9 diagnostic codes, including 850.11 (concussion with LOC of less than or equal to 30 minutes), V15.52 (V-code to be used with all TBI encounters), 907.0 (late effect of intracranial injury without skull fracture), 800–804 (various fractures of the skull), 850 (concussion), and 851–854 (various types of intracranial injuries).
[b] This diagnosis group contains all types of general medical exams, including V70.5 (postdeployment encounter).
[c] This diagnosis group is large and contains a number of TBI-related symptoms, including 780.93 (memory loss, NOS), 799.2 (nervousness, irritability, impulsiveness, etc.), and 780.5 and 780.52 (sleep disturbance and insomnia).

e.g., within psychological health, use of CAM for anxiety disorders was most prevalent, while CAM use for schizophrenia and other psychotic disorders was least prevalent.

Strengths and Limitations of Our Study

A major strength of this study is that it is based on data obtained from two different sources. Both the CAM survey and the MHS utilization data have strengths and weaknesses in terms of the breadth and validity of the contributed information. The CAM survey was specifically designed to provide an understanding of the use of CAM in the MHS through data not available from other sources. These data include the availability of CAM across the MHS, its use in terms of patient demand, conditions for which CAM is used, the documentation and coding of CAM use, provider credentialing and privileging, referrals and collaboration between CAM and conventional practitioners, and perceived effectiveness of the therapies. In particular, the CAM survey captures data on all CAM use, not just CAM therapies with existing procedure codes, and this facilitates a more comprehensive understanding of the availability of CAM services.

However, the survey data are limited because one person at each MTF who was tasked with gathering and reporting the data within a fairly short time frame collected them. We believe that each of these MTF-based POCs did their best. However, the data they were asked to report were not readily available in databases, or consistently captured in monitoring systems. In many cases, the information had to be collected from the impressions of a number of busy practitioners across the MTF. In addition, some of the questions asked for respondent perceptions or observations, and other questions may have been interpreted other than intended. Therefore, each respondent may have estimated answers based on slightly different response sets or sources of data.

On the other hand, the MHS health care utilization data are systematically collected and considered to be reasonably accurate. Health care providers are trained to report these data in a consistent manner because this information determines payment in many health care settings. While provider salaries are not directly linked to the provision of services in the MHS, there are productivity expectations, and documentation of provided services is the way productivity is determined. The utilization data report on the use of procedures, which can be applied to estimate numbers of patients and visits; in contrast, the CAM survey reports activities at an MTF-level. An additional advantage is that the utilization data were available for six years, making it possible to examine trends in CAM use over time.

However, MHS utilization data also have their limitations. The most important for our purposes is that many CAM therapies lack their own procedure codes; thus, use of the therapy can be documented only in the narrative section of the medical record and/or using more general procedure codes. The utilization data available to this study are also a bit dated (the most recent year available in our data set is 2013) and include only care given to Active Component service members. Finally, as noted above, the MHS utilization data cannot answer many of the questions needed for health care policy—e.g., regarding provider credentialing and privileging or the training they receive at the MTF. It can only report on prevalence of use of the CAM therapies for which procedure codes exist, the conditions and diagnoses for which they are used, and the types of providers delivering those therapies. Nevertheless, the MHS data provide an important complement to the information gleaned from the CAM survey.

Despite the limitations of the two data sources, the study benefited from the strengths and comparisons that were possible between answers given by each.

CHAPTER THREE

CAM Prevalence Across MTFs

This chapter describes the prevalence and types of CAM offered at the MTFs, the reasons MTFs give for offering (or not offering) CAM, the evidence used to justify their offerings, the CAM services to which other providers within the MTF most likely refer patients, and the CAM services MTFs are most interested in providing.

Out of the 133 MTFs responding to the survey, 83 percent of MTFs ($N = 110$) offer CAM services to their patients, 14 percent ($N = 18$) do not, and an additional 4 percent ($N = 5$) that currently do not offer them are planning to offer CAM services in the future. MTFs without CAM and no plans to offer CAM cite lack of provider availability and awareness or interest as the top reasons for not offering these services (see Figure 3.1), not lack of patient interest or worries about safety or efficacy.

Of the 115 MTFs that currently offer or plan to offer CAM, more than half endorsed one or more of five reasons for providing CAM: (1) as an adjunctive to chronic disease management; (2) to fulfill patient preference; (3) to promote wellness; (4) because of proven clinical

Figure 3.1
Reasons MTFs Do Not Offer CAM Services (N = 18)

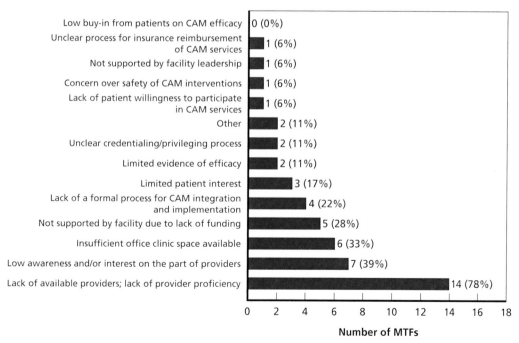

effectiveness; and (5) to fulfill provider request (see Figure 3.2). Half of MTFs also report that they offer CAM because it promotes cost savings.

Of the 110 MTFs that offer CAM, nine offer only one type of CAM, and two-thirds (73 MTFs) offer two to eight different types of CAM. In six MTFs, the CAM offerings are extensive, with 20 to 22 different types of CAM available (see Figure 3.3).

Six of the 23 MTFs that do not currently offer CAM services (including those planning to offer CAM services) recommend or refer patients to outside CAM services. For detail on the number of MTFs that refer patients or recommend care outside the MTF by type of CAM, see Appendix H, Table H.1.

Tables 3.1 and 3.2 show the number of CAM services offered by service branch and MTF size in terms of reported beneficiaries enrolled, respectively. The Air Force MTFs are less likely than the Army or Navy MTFs to offer any CAM services, but these relationships are not statistically significant. However, the Army MTFs are significantly more likely (p=0.0007) than the Air Force MTFs to offer 11 or more different CAM services. Because there are only three MTFs in the NCRMD, it is hard to generalize their findings. However, all three of these MTFs report CAM use. The Navy MTFs tend to offer CAM, but fewer types of CAM than are offered at Army MTFs.

The CAM survey data also show that, in general, larger MTFs (those reporting more beneficiaries enrolled) are both more likely to offer CAM services and offer a larger number of different types of CAM (see Table 3.2). MTFs reporting at least 25,000 beneficiaries are significantly more likely to both offer CAM (p=0.0003) and to offer 11 or more different types of CAM (p=0.0097) than are MTFs reporting fewer than 25,000 beneficiaries.

Figure 3.2
Reasons MTFs Offer or Plan to Offer CAM Services (N = 115)

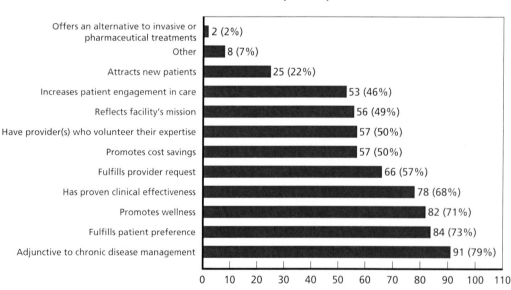

Figure 3.3
Number of CAM Services Provided in MTFs (*N* = 133)

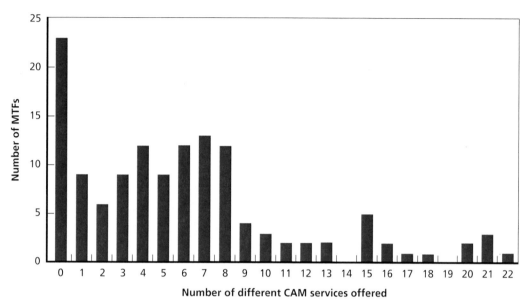

RAND RR1380-3.3

Table 3.1
Number of CAM Services Provided in MTFs by Branch of Service

Number of Different Types of CAM Services Provided	Air Force	Army	Navy	NCRMD
0 provided, 0 recommended outside the MTF	13 (18%)	2 (6%)	2 (7%)	0 (0%)
0 provided, ≥1 recommended outside the MTF	4 (6%)	1 (3%)	1 (4%)	0 (0%)
1–5	28 (39%)	7 (23%)	10 (37%)	0 (0%)
6–10	23 (32%)	10 (32%)	9 (33%)	2 (67%)
11–15	4 (6%)	6 (19%)	1 (4%)	0 (0%)
16–20	0 (0%)	2 (6%)	4 (15%)	0 (0%)
21–25	0 (0%)	3 (10%)	0 (0%)	1 (33%)
>25	0 (0%)	0 (0%)	0 (0%)	0 (0%)
Totals	72 (100%)	31 (100%)	27 (100%)	3 (100%)

Table 3.2
Number of CAM Services Provided in MTFs by MTF Size

Number of Different Types of CAM Services Provided	MTF Size by Reported Number of Beneficiaries Enrolled			
	<10,000	10,000 to 24,999	25, 000 to 99,999	>100,000
0 provided, 0 recommended outside the MTF	11 (27%)	6 (12%)	0 (0%)	0 (0%)
0 provided, ≥1 recommended outside the MTF	2 (5%)	4 (8%)	0 (0%)	0 (0%)
1–5	10 (24%)	21 (41%)	11 (35%)	0 (0%)
6–10	15 (37%)	15 (29%)	11 (35%)	2 (40%)
11–15	3 (7%)	4 (8%)	4 (13%)	0 (0%)
16–20	0 (0%)	1 (2%)	3 (10%)	2 (40%)
21–25	0 (0%)	0 (0%)	2 (6%)	1 (20%)
>25	0 (0%)	0 (0%)	0 (0%)	0 (0%)
Totals	41 (100%)	51 (100%)	31 (100%)	5 (100%)

Types of CAM Services Offered

Among the MTFs offering CAM services ($N = 110$), three-fourths offer stress management/relaxation therapy, and approximately two-thirds offer acupuncture (see Table 3.3). At least half of these MTFs offer progressive muscle relaxation, guided imagery, chiropractic services, and mindfulness meditation. At least one-fourth of MTFs offering CAM services provide diet therapy, nutritional supplements, biofeedback, acupressure, and yoga. Other CAM services were offered by fewer MTFs.

Many CAM services are offered in combination to patients to treat a single condition. Therefore, we allowed MTFs to report CAM services they offer (1) separately from other CAM services (alone), and/or (2) in combination with other CAM services. Table 3.4 presents the way MTFs report offering CAM services. We separated the combinations MTFs reported into those that included only CAM services within a general category of CAM (e.g., mind-body medicine; see Figure 1.1) and those that included CAM services from two or more categories of CAM (mixed combinations). No MTFs reported combinations that included only energy therapies or included only alternative or whole medical systems.

Each type of CAM service was reported as being used in combination with other CAM services by at least one MTF and as being used alone by at least two. As an example of how CAM use is reported, 83 MTFs reported that they offer stress management/relaxation therapy (Table 3.3). Forty-six of these MTFs reported this as a CAM service that was offered alone (i.e., separately from their other CAM service offerings), 42 MTFs reported that they offered this CAM service as part of a combined package of care with other mind-body medicine therapies, and 26 MTFs reported that they offered stress management/relaxation therapy in a mixed combination with other CAM services, including some that were not mind-body medicine.

Table 3.3
CAM Services Provided at MTFs, CAM Survey Data (*N* = 110 MTFs)

CAM Service	N	Percentage
Stress management/relaxation therapy	83	75
Acupuncture	76	69
Progressive muscle relaxation	64	58
Guided imagery	61	55
Chiropractic	60	55
Mindfulness meditation	56	51
Diet—special, diet therapy	52	47
Dietary/nutritional supplements	43	39
Biofeedback	39	35
Acupressure	30	27
Yoga	29	26
Other meditation	26	24
Massage therapy	22	20
Movement practices	16	15
Animal-assisted therapy	15	14
Hypnosis/hypnotherapy	15	14
Music therapy	15	14
Tai chi, qi gong	11	10
Dry needling	11	10
Osteopathic manipulative therapy	11	10
Aromatherapy	10	9
Mantram repetition meditation	10	9
Energy healing	9	8
Nontraditional spiritual practice	8	7
Traditional Chinese medicine	8	7
Other	7	6
Transcendental meditation	6	5
Herbal medicines	6	5
Hyperbaric oxygen therapy	6	5
Chelation therapy	0	0
Ayurveda	0	0
Homeopathy	0	0

Table 3.3—Continued

CAM Service	N	Percentage
Native American healing practices	0	0
Naturopathic medicine	0	0

NOTE: Because no MTFs offer chelation therapy, Ayurveda, homeopathy, Native American healing practices, or naturopathic medicine, these CAM services will not be discussed in the remainder of this report. "Other" CAM services included sensory deprivation (1), alpha stimulation (1), rehabilitative martial and henna arts (1), art therapy (1), trigger point therapy (2), and neurofeedback (1).

Note that MTFs could report separately on a CAM service's use alone and in one or more combinations of CAM therapies.

Stress management/relaxation therapies were not only the most common CAM service offered across MTFs, they are the most common type of CAM included in both the mind-body medicine combinations and the mixed combinations, with almost half of the MTFs offering this therapy only as part of a combination. In contrast, acupuncture is often offered alone, but it is also sometimes offered in combination. Acupuncture is offered by 76 MTFs; 62 MTFs report offering acupuncture alone, five offer it in other manipulative and body-based combinations, and 20 MTFs offer acupuncture in combination with a mixed set of CAM services.

At the bottom of Table 3.4, we report the number of combinations defined by MTFs and the number of unique MTFs reporting those types of combinations. MTFs that reported combinations tended to report more than one for all but the biologically based combinations. The average numbers of CAM services included in each type of combination were: 3.75 for mind-body medicine combinations; 2.20 for biologically based combinations; 2.1 for manipulative and body-based combinations; and 6.53 for mixed combinations (data not shown).

Overall, the reported combinations tended to be unique to an MTF. Nevertheless, there were some combinations that were repeated across MTFs. Within the mind-body medicine combinations, seven MTFs reported using the combination of guided imagery, mindfulness meditation, progressive muscle relaxation, and stress management/relaxation therapy. Five other MTFs reported using the combination of mindfulness meditation and stress management/relaxation therapy. Four MTFs reported using the combination of mindfulness meditation and progressive muscle relaxation, and four others reported using the combination of stress management/relaxation therapy, progressive muscle relaxation, guided imagery, mindfulness meditation, and other meditation. Of the ten MTFs that reported using biologically based combinations, eight were combinations of diet therapy and dietary supplements, and the other two added herbal medicine to this mix. Finally, of the six MTFs that reported using manipulative and body-based combinations, four offered acupuncture and acupressure in combination. Almost all other combinations were unique.

What Evidence Do MTFs Use When Deciding to Offer CAM Services?

The CAM survey asked MTFs about the type of evidence used to support the decision to provide a specific CAM service. Across commonly offered CAM services, 64 percent to 84 percent

Table 3.4
How CAM Services Are Offered and Reported at MTFs, CAM Survey Data

| CAM Service | Number of MTFs that report on this CAM therapy in each of these ways | | | | |
	Alone	Mind-Body Medicine Combination	Biologically Based Combination	Manipulative and Body-Based Combination	Mixed Combination
Mind-body medicine					
Stress management, relaxation therapy	46	42			26
Progressive muscle relaxation	32	35			21
Guided imagery	28	32			19
Mindfulness meditation	32	30			19
Biofeedback	28	7			10
Yoga	19	7			15
Other meditation	13	14			10
Animal-assisted therapy	12	3			1
Hypnosis/hypnotherapy	11	3			2
Music therapy	7	2			3
Aromatherapy	1	3			8
Mantram repetition meditation	6	5			6
Nontraditional spiritual practice	4	3			5
Transcendental meditation	4	2			4
Biologically based practices					
Diet—special, diet therapy	34		10		15
Dietary/nutritional supplements	31		10		9
Herbal medicines	2		2		3
Manipulative and body-based practices					
Acupuncture	62			5	20
Chiropractic	49			2	12
Acupressure	23			4	13
Massage therapy	14			1	15
Movement practices	8			1	9
Dry needling	7			2	5

Table 3.4—Continued

CAM Service	Alone	Number of MTFs that report on this CAM therapy in each of these ways			
		Mind-Body Medicine Combination	Biologically Based Combination	Manipulative and Body-Based Combination	Mixed Combination
Osteopathic manipulative therapy	11				2
Hyperbaric oxygen therapy	5			1	
Energy therapy					
Tai chi, qi gong	8				5
Energy healing	6				4
Whole medical systems					
Traditional Chinese medicine	6				7
Other					
Other	6				1
Summary statistics					
Sum of column	515				
Number of combinations		60	10	10	62
Number of unique MTFs		44	10	6	30

NOTE: "Other" included sensory deprivation (1), alpha stimulation (1), rehabilitative martial and henna arts (1), art therapy (1), trigger point therapy (2), and neurofeedback (1).

of MTFs said that their decisions were based on scientific evidence and/or clinical practice guidelines (see Figure 3.4). The majority of MTFs also report using experiential or anecdotal evidence, but it was used instead of scientific evidence or clinical practice guidelines in only a small number of cases (zero to 15 percent of the time) across these CAM services. Only rarely did MTFs report that no evidence was used in their decisions. Data on the types of evidence used to support the decisions to provide each type of CAM service appear in Appendix H, Table H.2.

CAM Use as Reported in the MHS Utilization Data

The MHS health care utilization data provide a different perspective on CAM use in MTFs. We examined the provision of CAM services documented in these utilization data for 2013, the most recent year for which we have data. Trends in the provision of CAM services were assessed using data from 2008 through 2013. As noted earlier, only a small number of CAM services have specific CPT or ICD-9 procedure codes that allow their use to be clearly docu-

Figure 3.4
Type of Evidence Used to Support the Decision to Provide CAM Services for the Ten Most Commonly Offered CAM Services

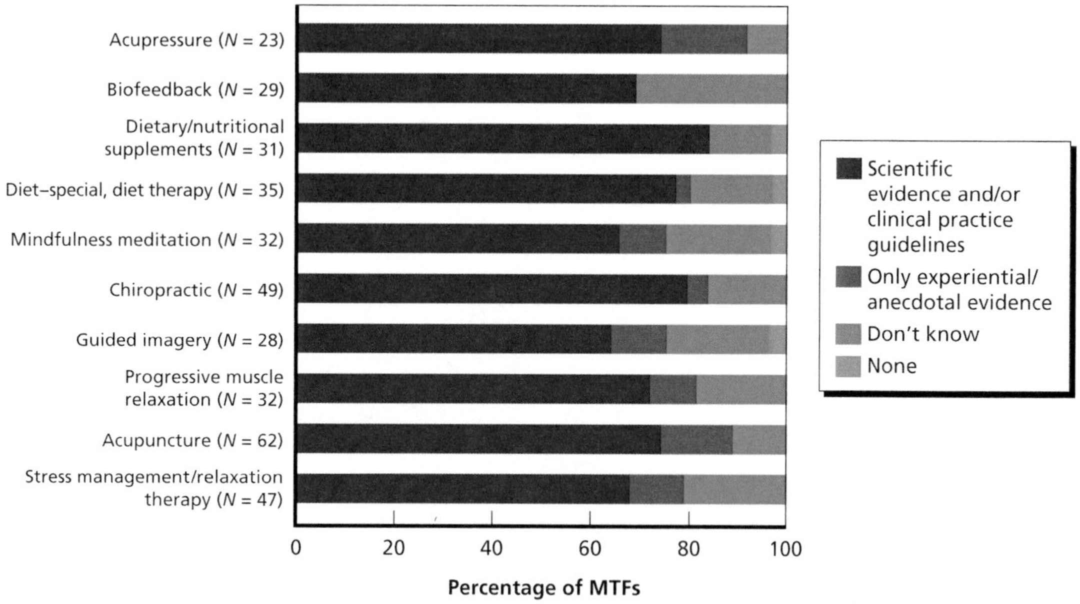

RAND *RR1380-3.4*

mented in the utilization data. These services are acupuncture, biofeedback, chiropractic, massage, and hypnosis/hypnotherapy (the codes we used for each are shown in Table 2.1).[1]

Across the 142 Army, Navy, Air Force and NCRMD MTFs in the MHS utilization database (see Appendix H, Table H.3), more than 90 percent ($N = 131$) had at least one instance of an outpatient CAM-specific code recorded in 2013, the most recent year for which we have these data, and more than 85 percent ($N = 121$) had at least ten instances of these codes being used. Given the different data sources and years, and the low nonresponse to the CAM survey, these figures are consistent with our finding that 83 percent of MTFs offer CAM.

The MHS utilization data allow us to go beyond the percentage of MTFs offering CAM to look at the relative frequency of patient-level CAM use. Table H.4 in Appendix H shows the frequency of use of the CAM therapies listed in Table 2.1 by year for 2008 through 2013, by inpatient and outpatient care, within MTFs, and by network providers and service branch.

Overall use of these CAM therapies has increased gradually over the 2008–2013 period (Figure 3.5 and Table H.4). Similar increases are seen for each therapy with the exception of massage.

According to the MHS utilization data, chiropractic is by far the most frequently used of the CAM services recorded in these data, followed by acupuncture and massage (see Figure 3.5). Thus, while the survey indicated that acupuncture is offered at a larger number of MTFs (69 percent), with chiropractic following at 55 percent (see Table 3.3), MHS utilization data indicate that more chiropractic procedures are delivered per year.

The majority of CAM use occurs in the MTF on an outpatient basis (i.e., direct outpatient care); CAM services are rarely provided in the inpatient setting (see Table H.4). Less than

---

[1]   Music therapy was identifiable by only one inpatient ICD-9 procedure code, which was rarely used. Therefore, we do not include music therapy in our discussion.

Figure 3.5
Frequency of CAM Use 2008 to 2013 by Type of CAM, MHS Utilization Data

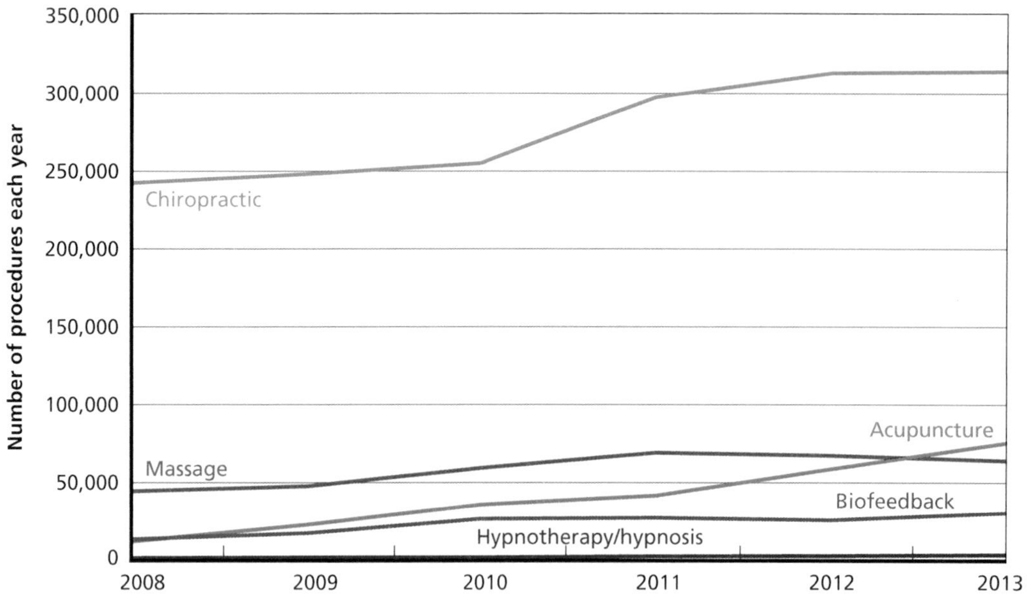

RAND RR1380-3.5

3 percent of outpatient use occurs outside the MTFs (i.e., purchased care). (This percentage is higher for massage—from 12 percent to 20 percent purchased outside the MTFs per year.) Many of the service members receiving CAM from civilian providers live far from an MTF. Sixty-six percent to 90 percent of purchased CAM care occurs in noncatchment areas—that is, areas 40 miles or more from the closest MTF.

The majority of CAM use, and most of the increase in use, has occurred in Army MTFs. CAM use was up by 109 percent in Army MTFs from 2008 to 2013. The increase in Navy MTFs was lower, but still substantial (52 percent). CAM use increased by only 3 percent in Air Force MTFs.

To What CAM Services Do Conventional Providers Refer Patients?

Among MTFs that offer CAM services, stress management/relaxation therapy was most often among the three most-commonly-referred-to CAM services by conventional health care providers (59 percent of MTFs offering CAM services), followed by acupuncture (57 percent), and chiropractic (48 percent) (see Figure 3.6).

The CAM survey also asked all MTFs ($N = 133$) to name the top three CAM services that they are most interested in offering, regardless of whether they currently offer them. The therapies most often mentioned were acupuncture (79 percent); chiropractic (63 percent); massage (38 percent); relaxation techniques (23 percent); nutrition and supplements consultation (22 percent); biofeedback (17 percent); yoga (14 percent); meditation (mindfulness, other; 12 percent); animal-assisted therapy (5 percent); and guided imagery (5 percent).

Figure 3.6
CAM Services Reported as Among Three Most Commonly Referred to by Conventional Health Care Providers at MTFs Offering CAM (N = 110 MTFs)

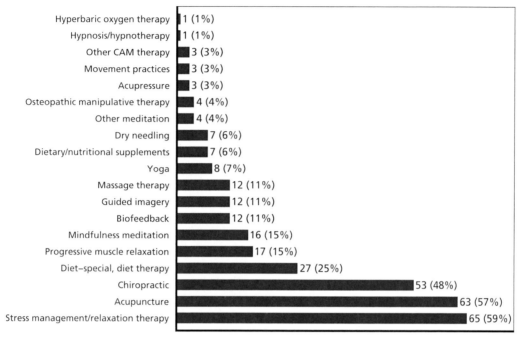

RAND RR1380-3.6

Prevalence of CAM: Key Points

- The majority of MTFs (83 percent) offer CAM services, usually one to eight different types.
- MTF providers may offer individual CAM services alone or in combination with other types of CAM treatments. The extent to which CAM is offered in combinations is substantial and varies by the type of CAM.
- Army MTFs are the most likely to offer a large number of CAM treatments. Larger MTFs are also more likely to offer CAM services and to provide a larger number of services.
- Most MTFs say they based the decision to offer CAM on a combination of scientific evidence and experiential and/or anecdotal evidence. However, the majority of MTFs do cite scientific evidence and/or clinical practice guidelines in their decisions.
- MTFs that do not offer CAM cite lack of available trained providers as the primary reason; few MTFs cite lack of patient interest or safety concerns.
- The majority of MTFs offering CAM services cite adjunctive use in chronic disease management, patient preference, wellness promotion, and clinical effectiveness as main reasons for offering CAM; half of MTFs cite cost savings.
- The majority of MTFs offer the following CAM services: stress management/relaxation therapy, acupuncture, progressive muscle relaxation, guided imagery, chiropractic, and mindfulness meditation. Acupuncture and chiropractic are the two CAM services that MTFs are most interested in offering.
- Acupuncture, chiropractic, and stress management/relaxation therapy are the CAM services to which conventional health care providers most commonly refer patients.
- While more MTFs report offering acupuncture, chiropractic services are the most used.

CHAPTER FOUR

Conditions and Diagnoses for Which CAM Is Used

MTFs that reported offering at least one CAM service were asked a more detailed set of questions about each CAM service. This and the next three chapters describe these results. This chapter focuses on the conditions for which each type of CAM is used, and each treatment's perceived patient adherence and effectiveness. In our discussion of the conditions for which CAM is used, we supplement data from the CAM survey with information from MHS utilization data.

How Is CAM Being Used?

The CAM survey asked about the reason or condition(s) for which each CAM service offered at the MTF is used. Conditions were grouped into four broad categories: chronic disease management; mental health; pain management; and miscellaneous conditions. Respondents could select multiple conditions for each type of CAM.

Figure 4.1 highlights the five conditions for which the use of CAM services was reported most often by MTFs. For each condition, we also present the five CAM services most commonly reported by MTFs as being used to treat it. The conditions represent a combination of pain and mental health conditions. Detailed data on the number of MTFs that reported using each CAM service for specific conditions are available in Appendix H, Table H.5.

Figure 4.1
Conditions for Which CAM Use Is Most Commonly Reported by MTFs and CAM Services Most Commonly Used for Each

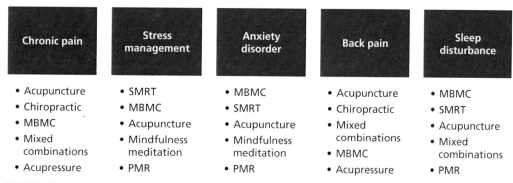

Chronic pain	Stress management	Anxiety disorder	Back pain	Sleep disturbance
• Acupuncture	• SMRT	• MBMC	• Acupuncture	• MBMC
• Chiropractic	• MBMC	• SMRT	• Chiropractic	• SMRT
• MBMC	• Acupuncture	• Acupuncture	• Mixed combinations	• Acupuncture
• Mixed combinations	• Mindfulness meditation	• Mindfulness meditation	• MBMC	• Mixed combinations
• Acupressure	• PMR	• PMR	• Acupressure	• PMR

NOTES: MBMC = mind-body medicine combinations; SMRT = stress management/relaxation therapy; PMR = progressive muscle relaxation.
RAND RR1380-4.1

According to 2013 MHS utilization data, nearly 90 percent of CAM (among services with existing codes) is used for chronic musculoskeletal pain (see Figure 4.2 and Table 4.1). The other categories of diagnoses or conditions for which CAM was used are psychological health and TBI and neurologic pathology.

As expected, chiropractic and massage are used almost exclusively (97 percent and 92 percent, respectively) for chronic musculoskeletal pain conditions (Table 4.1). The majority of acupuncture (62 percent) is also used for chronic musculoskeletal pain. In contrast, about two-thirds (65 percent) of hypnosis and 40 percent of biofeedback codes are used for psychological health conditions, and almost one-fifth of both acupuncture (19 percent) and hypnosis (17 percent) codes are used for TBI and neurologic pathology. Data by more-detailed diagnosis category (shown in Table 2.2 in Chapter Two) are found in Appendix H, Table H.6.

Do Patients Adhere to Treatment, and Is It Effective?

The CAM survey asked MTF respondents whether they thought patients adhered to CAM treatment and whether they thought CAM was effective.

Perceived Adherence

Respondents were asked to rank patient adherence as "high," "medium," and "low" (as well as "not applicable" and "don't know"). Figure 4.3 shows the reported levels of perceived patient adherence across the CAM services most often offered. Manipulative and body-based therapies, especially acupuncture and chiropractic, had higher rates of adherence than biologically based (dietary) interventions. For example, respondents in 61 percent of MTFs perceived that patients were highly likely to adhere to a prescribed chiropractic therapy, while 12 percent of MTF respondents reported patients as highly likely to adhere to prescribed diet therapy. This is likely because patients receive appointments for the first therapy and often have to practice the latter on their own. Detailed data on reported levels of perceived patient adherence for specific CAM services are available in Appendix H, Table H.7.

Figure 4.2
Types of Diagnoses for Which Outpatient CAM Was Used in 2013, MHS Utilization Data

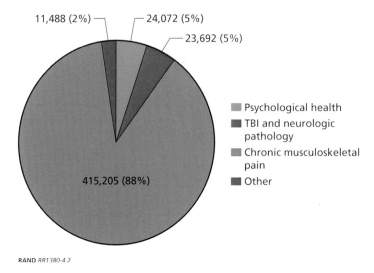

RAND RR1380-4.2

Table 4.1
Number of Outpatient CAM Services Used for Each Type of Diagnosis in 2013, MHS Utilization Data

Diagnosis Group Associated with Procedure	Acupuncture	Biofeedback	Chiropractic	Hypnosis/ Hypnotherapy	Massage	Totals
Chronic musculoskeletal pain	46,071	4,946	305,659	20	58,509	415,205
Psychological health	10,265	11,897	14	1,784	112	24,072
TBI and neurologic pathology	13,975	3,520	4,687	476	1,034	23,692
Other conditions[a]	4,433	9,523	3,572	482	3,697	21,707
Totals	74,744	29,886	313,932	2,762	63,352	484,676

[a] This grouping contains all other diagnoses for which these CAM therapies are used.

Figure 4.3
Reported Levels of Perceived Patient Adherence for CAM Services Most Frequently Offered by MTFs

		High Adherence (%)	Moderate Adherence (%)	Low Adherence (%)
Manipulative and body-based practices	Acupuncture (N = 62)	56	24	2
	Chiropractic (N = 49)	61	22	0
	Acupressure (N = 23)	22	26	4
Mind-body medicine	Stress management/relaxation therapy (N = 46)	24	33	0
	Mindfulness meditation (N = 32)	25	38	6
	Progressive muscle relaxation (N = 32)	31	34	3
	Guided imagery (N = 28)	18	46	0
Biologically based practices	Diet therapy (N = 33)	12	39	15
	Dietary supplements (N = 31)	13	45	3

NOTE: N = the number of MTFs that offer the specific CAM service and that reported on it alone. The percentages for the "not applicable" and "don't know" responses are not shown.
RAND RR1380-4.3

Perceived Effectiveness

The CAM survey asked about the types of benefits for which each CAM service showed "the most success per patient and provider report." Figure 4.4 highlights the five benefits MTFs most often reported and the five CAM services most commonly reported as showing that benefit. Detailed data are provided in Appendix H, Table H.8.

When a respondent reported reduced pain; reduced symptoms of depression, anxiety, or PTSD; or improved sleep for a particular CAM service, the CAM survey then asked whether there had been "an observed reduction" in patients' use of medications for these problems. For the ten CAM services reported most often as improving pain, depression, anxiety, PTSD, or sleep disturbance, Figure 4.5 depicts the percentage of MTFs that reported reductions in any medication used to treat these conditions. Acupuncture and chiropractic were the two CAM services most often associated with a reduction in medication. Detailed data for specific CAM services are presented in Appendix H, Table H.9.

Use of CAM in MTFs—Key Points

- MTFs report that CAM services are most often used to treat chronic pain, stress, anxiety, back pain, and sleep disturbance.
- The CAM services most often used for these conditions are acupuncture (all five conditions), combinations of mind-body medicine therapies (all five), acupressure (both pain conditions), chiropractic (both pain conditions), progressive muscle relaxation (three psychological health conditions), and stress management/relaxation therapy (three psychological health conditions).
- The MHS utilization data also indicate that most CAM therapies are used for chronic musculoskeletal pain, with chiropractic services representing almost all of this care.
- Reported rates of patient adherence tended to be higher for manipulative and body-based therapies (e.g., acupuncture and chiropractic) than for biologically based (dietary) interventions. This could be because patients often have to practice the latter on their own.
- Effectiveness per provider and patient report of success was most often reported by MTFs for acupuncture, mind-body medicine combinations, and stress management/relaxation therapy for improved quality of life, reduced pain, reduced stress, reduced anxiety, and improved patient satisfaction. Chiropractic was one of the most commonly used CAM therapies for improved quality of life, reduced pain, and improved patient satisfaction, while mindfulness meditation was one of the most commonly reported CAM therapies for reduced stress and anxiety.
- Acupuncture and chiropractic services were reported most frequently by MTFs as resulting in reduction of medication use.

Figure 4.4
Most Common Benefits from CAM Services per Patient and Provider Report and the CAM Services Most Often Reported as Showing That Benefit

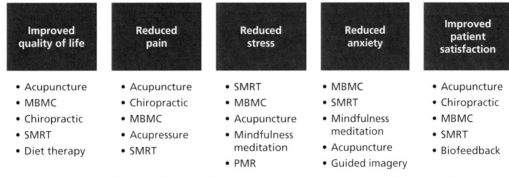

Improved quality of life	Reduced pain	Reduced stress	Reduced anxiety	Improved patient satisfaction
• Acupuncture	• Acupuncture	• SMRT	• MBMC	• Acupuncture
• MBMC	• Chiropractic	• MBMC	• SMRT	• Chiropractic
• Chiropractic	• MBMC	• Acupuncture	• Mindfulness meditation	• MBMC
• SMRT	• Acupressure	• Mindfulness meditation	• Acupuncture	• SMRT
• Diet therapy	• SMRT	• PMR	• Guided imagery	• Biofeedback

NOTES: MBMC = mind-body medicine combinations; SMRT = stress management/relaxation therapy; PMR = progressive muscle relaxation.
RAND RR1380-4.4

Figure 4.5
Reported Reduction in Medication Use Among Users of CAM Services

Top 10 CAM Therapies in Which Improvements for Pain, Depression, Anxiety, PTSD, and Sleep Were Most Often Reported	Percentage of MTFs That Reported Related Reduction in Medication Use (%)
Acupuncture (N = 59)	61
Chiropractic (N = 46)	59
Mind-body combinations (N = 41)	37
Stress management/relaxation therapy (N = 39)	21
Mindfulness meditation (N = 29)	34
Progressive muscle relaxation (N = 28)	32
Guided imagery (N = 26)	27
Biofeedback (N = 22)	41
Acupressure (N = 21)	43
Dietary/nutritional supplements (N = 16)	13

NOTE: N = The number of MTFs that reported offering that particular therapy and using it alone—i.e., not in combination with other CAM services—and named that therapy as one that showed benefits for pain, depression, anxiety, PTSD, and/or sleep per patient and provider report.
RAND RR1380-4.5

CHAPTER FIVE

Demand for CAM Services at MTFs

We estimated patient demand for CAM in three ways. We first examine MTF reports of how often providers receive requests from patients for CAM services. We then report on "fulfilled demand"—that is, the estimated number of patient encounters per month that MTFs report for each type of CAM offered, and compare these estimates with the number of CAM procedures and visits recorded in the MHS health care utilization data. Finally, we present MTF reports of wait lists for CAM services (i.e., "unmet demand").

How Often Do Patients Request CAM?

We asked MTFs to report how often providers received requests from patients for CAM services (Figure 5.1). Forty percent of MTFs reported that their providers received such requests "often" (36 percent) or "always" (4 percent). Almost one-quarter of MTFs reported rarely (20 percent) or never (2 percent) receiving patient requests for CAM services. The remaining 44 percent of MTFs sometimes received requests from patients. MTFs that offer CAM services were more likely to often/always receive requests for CAM (45 percent) than MTFs not offering CAM (13 percent). Half of the MTFs that do not offer CAM and have no plans to do so reported that requests for CAM occurred "rarely." The frequency of patient requests for

Figure 5.1
Frequency of Providers' Receipt of Requests from Patients for CAM Services (N = 133)

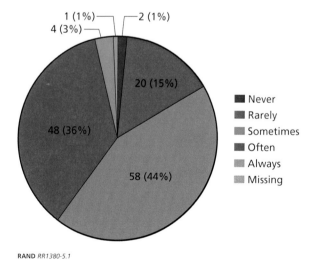

1 (1%) — 2 (1%)
4 (3%)
20 (15%)
48 (36%)
58 (44%)

- ■ Never
- ■ Rarely
- Sometimes
- ■ Often
- Always
- Missing

RAND RR1380-5.1

MTFs planning to offer CAM showed a distribution similar to the distribution among MTFs currently offering CAM.

How Often Are CAM Services Used?

We assessed the fulfilled demand for CAM services in MTFs by asking for an estimate of the number of patient encounters per month for each CAM service offered in MTFs. Respondents were asked to select one of the following categories: fewer than 50; 51 to 100; 101 to 150; 151 to 200; 201 to 500; or more than 500. There is substantial variation—both across type of CAM and across MTFs—in the monthly number of patient encounters in which these CAM services are used alone (Figure 5.2). For example, about two-thirds of MTFs offering acupuncture, stress management/relaxation therapy, progressive muscle relaxation, biofeedback and acupressure reported fewer than 50 patient encounters per month for these services. In contrast, only 10 percent of MTFs offering chiropractic reported fewer than 50 patient encounters per month, and almost 20 percent reported more than 500 chiropractic patient encounters per month. In addition, MTFs reported on 17 different combinations of CAM services with more than 500 patient encounters per month (Table 5.1; each column represents a combination of CAM services). Detailed data for the MTF estimates of current number of patient encounters per month are available in Appendix H, Table H.10.

Figure 5.2
Patient Encounters per Month in MTFs for Most Commonly Offered CAM Services (*N* = 110)

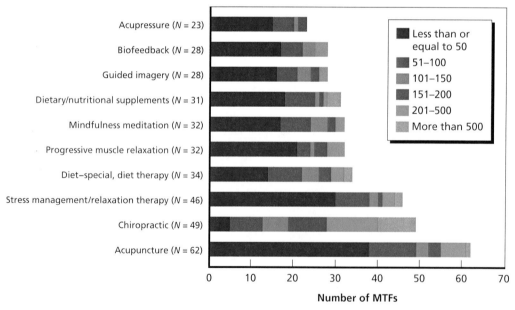

RAND *RR1380-5.2*

Table 5.1
CAM Service Combinations that MTFs Reported as Having >500 Patient Encounters per Month

CAM Service	Mixed Combinations										Mind-Body Combinations					Manipulative and Body-Based Combination	Biologically Based Combination
	1	2	3	4	5	6	7	8	9	10	1	2	3	4	5		
Mind-Body Medicine																	
Stress management, relaxation therapy	X	X	X	X	X	X	X	X			X	X	X	X	X		
Progressive muscle relaxation	X	X	X	X	X	X		X			X	X	X	X			
Biofeedback	X		X		X	X	X	X		X	X			X			
Mindfulness meditation	X	X	X	X		X					X	X	X				
Yoga	X		X	X	X		X	X	X			X					
Guided imagery	X	X			X	X	X		X								
Other meditation	X		X	X		X					X						
Aromatherapy		X		X	X												
Hypnosis/ hypnotherapy		X			X												
Animal assisted therapy	X																
Transcendental meditation	X																
Mantram repetition meditation			X														
Music therapy		X															
Nontraditional spiritual practice								X									
Biologically Based Practices																	
Diet—special, diet therapy		X	X	X		X	X										X
Dietary/nutritional supplements		X	X	X		X											X
Herbal medicines		X															
Manipulative and Body-Based Practices																	
Acupuncture	X	X	X	X	X	X	X	X								X	
Massage therapy	X	X	X	X	X	X	X		X								
Chiropractic	X	X	X	X	X		X	X								X	
Acupressure	X	X	X	X	X	X		X									

Table 5.1—Continued

CAM Service	Mixed Combinations										Mind-Body Combinations					Manipulative and Body-Based Combination	Biologically Based Combination
	1	2	3	4	5	6	7	8	9	10	1	2	3	4	5		
Movement practices					X	X	X										
Dry needling																X	
Osteopathic manipulative therapy									X								
Energy Therapies																	
Tai chi, qi gong	X		X														
Energy healing	X																
Alternative or Whole Medical Systems																	
Traditional Chinese medicine	X	X	X	X			X										

NOTE: Each column represents one MTF-defined combination of CAM services where estimated patient encounters per month were >500. There were 10 mixed combinations, 5 mind-body combinations, 1 manipulative and body-based combination, and 1 biologically-based combination that each were estimated by an MTF to have >500 patient encounters per month. The X's in each column identify the CAM services that made up each combination.

We also estimated the total number of patient encounters for each type of CAM service across all MTFs by assigning a number to each of the patient encounter categories assessed, and then summing these numbers across all MTFs that offer that type of CAM service. The numbers assigned to each patient encounter category correspond generally to the midpoint of each range for the main estimate and to the bottom and top of each range for the low and high estimates, respectively.[1] Across all types of CAM services and all MTFs, the total estimated number of patient encounters was almost 76,000 (45,500 to 106,000) per month. However, utilization varies widely across type of CAM service. For example, chiropractic and mind-body medicine combinations are among the CAM services with the highest estimated number of encounters; transcendental meditation and aromatherapy are among the CAM services with the lowest estimated number of encounters.

Figure 5.3 shows the five CAM services with the most and least patient encounters per month. Figure 5.4 shows the estimated total frequency of patient encounters per month across all MTFs by specific CAM services. Detailed data for the number of patient encounters per month for CAM services are available in Appendix H, Table H.10.

---

[1]   For the main estimate, the following numbers were assigned to each category of patient encounters: fewer than 50→25; 51–100→75; 101–150→125; 151–200→175; 201–500→350; more than 500→750. For the low estimate, we used the low end of each range (e.g., zero for the first category); for the high estimate, we used the high end of each range and used 1,000 for the more-than-500 category.

Figure 5.3
Five CAM Services Offered in MTFs With the Most and Least Patient Encounters per Month

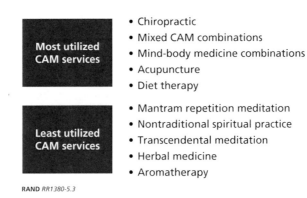

Most utilized CAM services

- Chiropractic
- Mixed CAM combinations
- Mind-body medicine combinations
- Acupuncture
- Diet therapy

Least utilized CAM services

- Mantram repetition meditation
- Nontraditional spiritual practice
- Transcendental meditation
- Herbal medicine
- Aromatherapy

RAND RR1380-5.3

Figure 5.4
Estimated Frequency of Patient Encounters per Month Across All MTFs, by Specific CAM Services

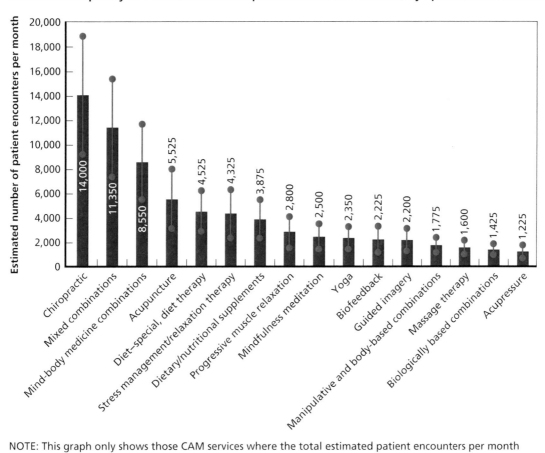

NOTE: This graph only shows those CAM services where the total estimated patient encounters per month across MTFs is greater than 1,000. The solid bars represent estimates based on the midpoint of the encounter ranges, while the lines ending in red dots represent estimates based on the lower and upper bounds of the ranges. The data labels are the values for the midpoint estimates.
RAND RR1380-5.4

Comparing Estimated Patient Encounters and Actual Patient Visits

We compared the estimated number of patient encounters from the CAM survey with the 2013 outpatient MTF-based (direct care) MHS utilization data (see Table 5.2). In general, the number of procedures by CAM type is roughly equivalent to the number of patient visits (patient visits were calculated following the assumption that all procedures for one patient on one day equal a visit). The exception is acupuncture. On average, providers recorded 1.67 acupuncture procedures per visit. The CPT codes for acupuncture are designed so that one procedure code is used for the first 15 minutes of treatment, and another is used for a subsequent 15 minutes, if needed. Therefore, it looks like about two-thirds of the visits for acupuncture utilize a second 15 minutes. However, although the massage therapy CPT code (97124) also covers 15 minutes of treatment, the number of massage procedures exactly equals the number of massage visits, which could mean that all MTF-based massages are limited to 15 minutes, or could reflect some other coding rule in the MHS. The second-to-last column in Table 5.2 shows that on average, patients using these five CAM services receive three to six visits per year.

Table 5.2
Patient Procedures and Visits from MHS Utilization Data Compared with Estimated Patient Encounters from CAM Survey

Service	From 2013 MHS Outpatient Direct Health Care Utilization Data					Estimated Patient Encounters per Year from CAM Survey[b]
	Number of Procedures	Estimated Number of Visits[a]	Average Number of Procedures per Visit	Number of Unique Patients	Average Number of Visits per Patient	
Acupuncture	74,311	44,461	1.67	11,932	3.73	66,300 (36,000–96,600)
Biofeedback	28,044	27,611	1.02	7,276	3.79	26,700 (13,800–39,600)
Chiropractic	313,438	299,669	1.05	55,843	5.37	168,000 (111,000–225,000)
Hypnosis/ hypnotherapy	2,722	2,600	1.05	645	4.03	4,500 (1,200–7,800)
Massage	55,801	55,757	1	15,464	3.61	19,200 (12,000–26,400)
Any of the above	474,316	408,847	1.16	79,006	5.17	—
All or any outpatient direct care	45,193,750	18,885,329	2.39	1,919,676	9.84	—
CAM percentage	1%	2%	—	4%	—	—

[a] Procedures that happen on the same day for the same patient are assumed to make up one patient visit.

[b] For comparison, reported here are the MTFs' estimates of patient encounters per month for each type of CAM multiplied by 12 to generate annual numbers. MTFs reported estimates of the number of patient encounters using six range categories, and the following numbers were used to represent each category in the calculations here: fewer than 50→25; 51–100→75; 101–150→125; 151–200→175; 201–500→350; more than 500→750. For the low and high estimates (in parentheses), the lower end (e.g., zero for fewer than 50) and higher end (1,000 for more than 500) of each range was used.

The data shown in Table 5.2 allow us to determine the proportion of total outpatient direct care that CAM represents. The five CAM procedures shown in Table 5.1 constitute 1 percent of all procedures across all MTFs and 2 percent of total visits. One out of every 25 patients (4 percent) with any outpatient direct care at the MTF in fiscal year 2013 received at least one of these five CAM services.

Comparison of the second and the last columns of Table 5.1—i.e., the number of actual visits (MHS) versus estimated patient encounters (CAM survey)—shows that the estimates of patient encounters provided by our respondents at the MTFs are generally reasonable—i.e., not orders of magnitude off. We would not expect the figures to match exactly for several reasons. First, the MHS utilization data are for fiscal year 2013, and the CAM survey was fielded in 2015. Second, the survey numbers could be higher because the utilization data cover only care for active military and activated Guard and Reserve component service members, not all care at the MTF. Third, the survey numbers could be lower because patient encounters for a portion of these CAM therapies could have been counted in the estimates given for the CAM combinations defined by respondents (see Table 3.4), i.e., combinations of CAM therapies that tended to be offered together to patients by the same practitioner.

The mixed combinations group was itself estimated to account for a total of 11,350 patient encounters per month (i.e., 136,200 per year). This patient encounter estimate cannot be allocated accurately across the CAM therapies included in the combinations because there is no information on how often each therapy in the combinations was actually used. We also cannot be sure that, if a number of CAM therapies were offered during a single visit, they were all recorded by CPT code when one was available.

The sum of the patient encounter estimates for the five CAM services shown in Table 5.1 comprises approximately 30 percent (24,400/76,000) of patient encounters across all CAM types (see Figure 5.4). If we assume that the 408,847 visits for the five CAM services shown in Table 5.1 make up 30 percent of all CAM visits, we can estimate total CAM visits at 1,362,823 (408,847/0.30). Therefore, CAM visits are estimated to make up approximately 7 percent (1,362,823/18,885,329) of total outpatient MTF visits.

Are Patients Waiting for CAM Services?

We assessed unmet demand for CAM services in MTFs using the CAM survey. Respondents were asked to estimate the number of patients on a waiting list for each CAM service provided at the MTF. Figure 5.5 shows the number of patients on a waiting list in the MTFs offering the specific type of CAM for the ten most commonly offered CAM services. The extent to which wait lists exist varies by the type of CAM, as does awareness about whether wait lists exist. Less than 25 percent of MTFs reported having wait lists for guided imagery, diet therapy, and nutritional supplements; when wait lists did exist, they almost always consisted of fewer than 40 people. Twenty-five percent to 35 percent of MTFs reported waiting lists for acupressure, biofeedback, mindfulness mediation, progressive muscle relaxation, and relaxation therapy; when wait lists existed, they usually consisted of fewer than 40 people. In contrast, approximately 45 percent of MTFs reported a wait list for chiropractic and acupuncture, with one-third to one-half of the wait lists consisting of more than 40 people. Fourteen percent (guided imagery) to 44 percent (diet therapy) of MTFs reported uncertainty about whether a wait list existed for CAM services. Detailed data for the number of patients on the waiting list for specific CAM services are available in Appendix H, Table H.11.

Figure 5.5
Number of Patients on a Wait List at MTFs for Commonly Offered CAM Services

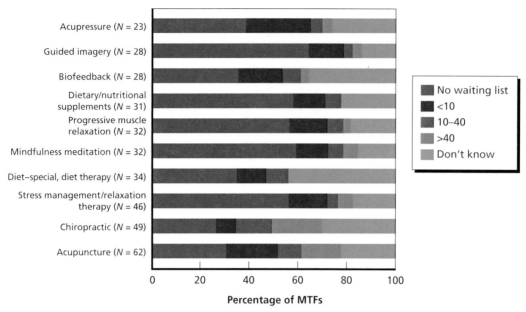

RAND RR1380-5.5

Demand for CAM: Key Points

- Almost 40 percent of MTFs report that their providers receive requests from patients for CAM services "often" or "always." Another 44 percent of MTFs report that their providers sometimes receive these requests. These requests happen most often in MTFs that offer CAM.
- Based on the CAM survey, almost 76,000 patient encounters per month are estimated to occur for CAM services. More than half of the total is made up of acupuncture, chiropractic, mixed CAM combinations, and mind-body medicine combinations.
- Comparing the estimates of patient visits from the CAM survey with the MHS utilization data indicates that the MTF-based estimates are reasonable.
- On average, patients receive three to six visits per year for hypnosis/hypnotherapy, massage, acupuncture, biofeedback, and chiropractic.
- Use of any of these five CAM therapies constitutes 1 percent of total MTF-based outpatient procedures, 2 percent of MTF-based outpatient visits, and 4 percent of unique MTF outpatients. The visit proportion across all CAM types is roughly 7 percent.
- Among MTFs offering seven of the ten most common types of CAM, fewer than 30 percent reported having a wait list, and wait lists were usually short when they did exist. In contrast, almost half of MTFs reported having wait lists for acupuncture and chiropractic, and one-third to one-half of these wait lists contained more than 40 patients. Depending on the type of CAM, it was unclear whether a wait list existed for 14 percent to 44 percent of MTFs.

CHAPTER SIX

Practitioners Who Provide CAM at MTFs

Both the data from the CAM survey and MHS utilization data provide information about the providers who deliver CAM at MTFs. In this chapter, we first focus on the types of practitioners providing each type of CAM, and then, from the CAM survey, we describe the clinical settings in which they practice, their collaboration with conventional medical practitioners and common sources for referrals to CAM. We then address CAM provider credentialing and privileging and the types of training that the MTFs provide these practitioners from the CAM survey.

Who Delivers CAM, and How Much Time Do They Spend?

Figure 6.1 shows the number and proportion of full-time equivalents (FTEs) attributable to each type of provider for all CAM services provided in all MTFs using the CAM survey data. Physicians (MDs/DOs of various specialty types) spend the most time providing CAM services (352.5 FTEs).[1] Clinical psychologists follow as a close second (316.5 FTEs); the third most common group delivering CAM services is licensed social workers (190 FTEs). These three types of providers are responsible for more than half of the total 1,555 FTEs of staff time devoted to CAM (see Appendix H, Table H.12A).

CAM is provided less frequently by contractors or volunteers—the other category offered in the survey instrument. Clinical psychologists are the most common group providing CAM as contractors or volunteers. Detailed data on provider FTEs for all CAM services provided at the MTF by MTF staff and contractors/volunteers are contained in Appendix H, Tables H.12A and H.12B, respectively.

We also used the 2013 MHS utilization data to examine the types of providers who provide outpatient CAM services at MTFs (see Table 6.1). The types of providers are listed in decreasing order of their overall provision of CAM. The *Physicians* (MD/DO) group includes physicians of any specialty. The *Other* group includes MHS-designated provider types, such as optometry, audiology, pharmacists, lab and pathology technicians, corpsmen, medical chemists, and students. The *Behavioral Health* group includes provider types, such as clinical psychologists, master's-level social workers, and behavioral technicians. The *Nursing* group includes registered nurses, nurse practitioners, nurse anesthetists, nurse midwives, and licensed practical nurses.

---

[1] This is equivalent to 352 physicians across the MTFs devoting their full time, plus one physician devoting half time, to the delivery of CAM services over the year.

Figure 6.1
Number of FTEs Accounted for by MTF Staff and Contractors/Volunteers of Different Provider Types, All CAM Services Provided in MTFs

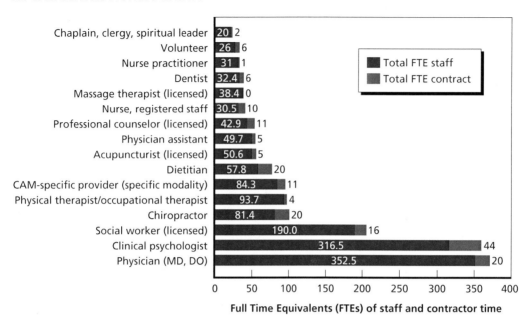

NOTE: This chart shows all provider types who are estimated to spend a total of >20 FTEs of staff and provider time delivering CAM across the MTFs.
RAND RR1380-6.1

As Table 6.1 highlights, more than two-thirds of visits across these five CAM therapies are being provided by chiropractors who are generally providing chiropractic manipulative services. However, chiropractors are also responsible for about 30 percent of the massage procedures. Physicians of all specialties are the next largest group providing CAM (11 percent of procedures), most often acupuncture. Indeed, physicians provided half of the acupuncture services in 2013. As expected given their training, behavioral health providers (e.g., psychologists, social workers, counselors) provide the vast majority (94 percent) of services for hypnotherapy, and more than half (59 percent) of those for biofeedback. The *Other* provider group provided more than half of the massage episodes in 2013. Within this group, the provider type called "corpsman/technician" provided the majority of CAM use, mostly massage. Dentists provided only acupuncture and not very frequently.

CAM Clinical Settings and Integration of CAM into MTFs

We asked how CAM services are integrated into the existing structure of MTFs that offered at least one CAM service. Specifically, we asked about the clinical settings in which CAM services are offered at the MTF, the level of collaboration between CAM and conventional providers, and the source of referrals for CAM services. Figure 6.2 highlights the findings on clinical settings. Most CAM is provided in outpatient MTF settings, usually outpatient primary care and behavioral health.

The majority of 110 MTFs (64 percent) that offer CAM do not have an integrative medicine or CAM-specialty clinic. CAM is offered in such clinics in only about one-third of

Table 6.1
Numbers of Outpatient CAM Procedures Delivered by Different Types of Providers in MTFs, by Type of CAM in 2013 MHS Utilization Data

Appointment Provider Specialty Code	Acupuncture	Biofeedback	Chiropractic	Hypnosis/ Hypnotherapy	Massage	Totals
Chiropractors	6,250	5	303,468	0	15,460	325,183
Physicians (MD/DO)	38,460	1,882	9,471	71	339	50,223
Other (e.g., students, optometry, audiology, pharmacists, lab techs, corpsman, pathology techs, medical chemists)	8,290	7,072	248	101	28,975	44,686
Physical and occupational therapy	14,586	1,773	32	0	10,978	27,369
Behavioral health (includes clinical psychologists, master's-level social workers, behavioral technicians)	4,458	16,452	0	2,546	0	23,456
Nursing (includes registered nurses, nurse practitioners, nurse anesthetists, nurse midwives, licensed practical nurses)	1,379	692	1	4	8	2,084
Physicians assistants	740	168	218	0	41	1,167
Dentists	148	0	0	0	0	148
Totals	74,311	28,044	313,438	2,722	55,801	474,316

MTFs. Integrative medicine/health clinics are more common (23 percent of MTFs offering CAM) than CAM specialty clinics (12 percent). The offer of CAM in these clinics seems to be only marginally related to MTF size: the smallest MTFs, in terms of estimated beneficiaries enrolled, are about as likely to offer CAM in an integrative medicine clinic as the larger MTFs, but only half as likely to offer CAM in a CAM specialty clinic.

It is fairly rare (8 percent of the 110 MTFs that offer CAM) that CAM providers do not interface with conventional medical providers. The open discussion of mutual patients happens in almost 60 percent of MTFs, and mutual referrals happen in 44 percent. In 17 percent of MTFs, conventional providers are the CAM providers. Primary care is one of the top three referral sources in almost all (95 percent) MTFs that offer CAM, and referrals from behavioral health providers (78 percent) and self-referrals (62 percent) are also common.

For those MTFs reporting that they have an integrative medicine or CAM specialty clinic, we asked about the duration of the clinic's existence and its current funding source. Of the 38 MTFs with a CAM or integrative health/medicine clinic, nearly 20 percent ($N = 7$) had been around for one year or less, slightly more than one-third had been around for two to four years ($N = 14$), less than 10 percent had been around for five to seven years ($N = 3$), and slightly more than one-third had been around for more than seven years ($N = 14$). About

Figure 6.2
Clinical Settings in Which CAM Services Are Offered in MTFs (*N* = 110)

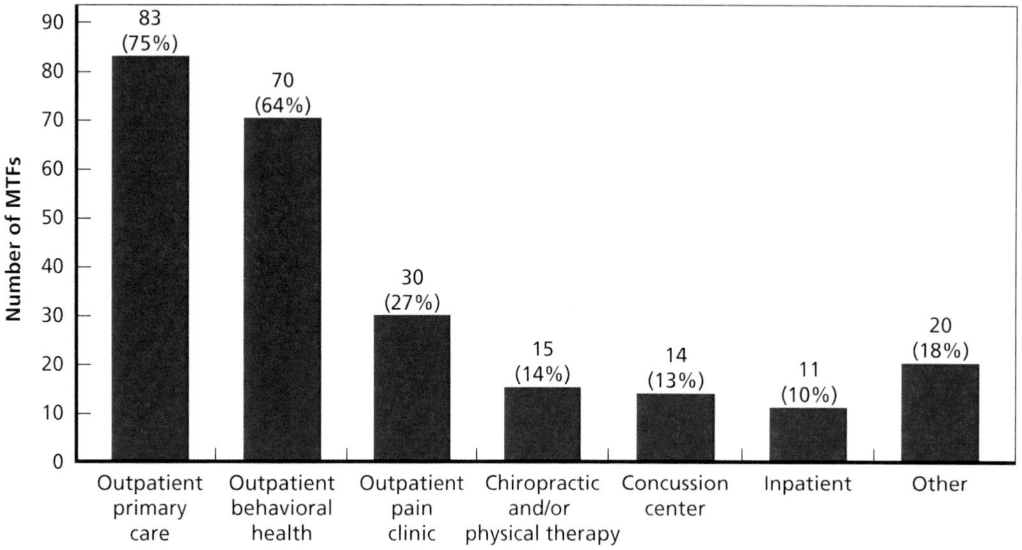

NOTE: The "other" group here includes the responses given by fewer than 10 MTFs each, including wellness centers (5 MTFs), family and children programs (4 MTFs), and rehabilitation centers (3 MTFs).
RAND RR1380-6.2

85 percent of CAM or integrative health and medicine clinics were funded as part of the MTF's overhead. Other sources of funding included an Interdisciplinary Pain Management Center (18 percent), Wounded, Ill, and Injured funding (5 percent), and other sources (5 percent).

How Much Is Invested in CAM Annually?

We used the FTE estimates provided by the MTFs to generate a rough estimate of the total annual (labor-only) investment in CAM services across the MHS. Our "back-of-the-envelope" approach entailed estimating the investment in CAM based on time spent by different types of practitioners in providing CAM services. We made this estimate for each CAM service by multiplying the total number of provider FTEs spent delivering that type of CAM service across MTFs over the past year (from Figure 6.1 and Table H.12A and H.12B) by the corresponding estimate of the average salary for each category of provider. These dollar amounts are then summed across provider types to generate a total labor investment estimate for each type of CAM service and summed across CAM services to generate a total labor investment estimate by provider type.

The total annual labor investment across all CAM is equivalent to the sum across the estimates for each type of CAM service or for each provider type. We had separate estimates for MTF staff and contractor or volunteer time, so we were able to estimate the investment in CAM for each group.

As described earlier, MTFs reported FTEs associated with each CAM service. Salary estimates are based on the average (across steps) 2015 Office of Personnel Management base salary levels for each General Schedule (GS) pay grade.[2] The GS grade for each type of provider was determined using the Fully Automated System for Classification and the GS grade and average salary assumed by provider type can be seen in Appendix H, Table H.13. We have assumed equivalent pay rates for MTF staff and contractors.

There were several provider types allowed in the data collection instrument that do not have obvious GS grade classifications. These were CAM-specific providers (trained and/or licensed in a specific modality—other than acupuncturists, chiropractors, and massage therapists), volunteers, and "other." We used the average GS grade-based salaries across the other provider types for these categories. In total these three provider types accounted for less than 7 percent of the total dollar investment, so this assumption has a minimal impact on our overall estimate.

We estimate that the total MHS labor investment in CAM for 2015 was approximately $112.7 million. Of this, the majority ($100.8 million) is MTF staff time. This figure likely understates the total investment in CAM for at least two reasons: (1) We used base GS salaries (e.g., salaries that do not contain adjustments for locality pay, nor do they include the value of benefits) to value the FTEs; and (2) we did not include the cost of facility space (e.g., the treatment rooms) and materials (e.g., acupuncture needles).

Figure 6.3 shows the estimated investment by CAM type and by provider type for the ten types of CAM with the greatest investment and the ten practitioner types through which the greatest investment in CAM is being made, respectively. Estimates for the full list of provider and CAM types are shown in Appendix H, Tables H.13 and H.14, respectively.

Figure 6.3
Estimates of MHS Labor Investment in CAM by CAM Type and Provider Type

MHS Labor Investment Top 10 CAM Types	MHS Labor Investment Top 10 Provider Types
Mixed combinations ($17.4M)	Physician (MD/DO) ($31.3M)
Acupuncture ($17.4M)	Clinical psychologist ($25.5M)
Stress management/relaxation therapy ($13.5M)	Social worker (licensed) ($11.0M)
Mind-body medicine combinations ($9.2M)	Chiropractor ($7.1M)
Dietary/nutritional supplements ($6.8M)	CAM-specific provider (trained and/or licensed in specific modality) ($5.3M)
Diet–special, diet therapy ($6.0M)	Physical therapist/occupational therapist ($4.3M)
Progressive muscle relaxation ($5.9M)	Acupuncturist (licensed) ($3.9M)
Guided imagery ($5.7M)	Dietitian ($3.8M)
Chiropractic ($5.0M)	Physician assistant ($3.2M)
Biofeedback ($4.2M)	Professional counselor (licensed) ($2.9M)

RAND *RR1380-6.3*

---

[2]   This table of salaries, accessed on December 11, 2015, can be found on the Office of Personnel Management website (OPM, 2015).

Who Is Responsible for Credentialing and Privileging CAM Providers?

We asked each MTF about the entities responsible for reviewing and approving the credentialing and privileging of providers of CAM services in MTFs. Figure 6.4 shows the distribution of this responsibility across various entities for the ten CAM services most frequently offered by MTFs. Among MTFs offering the CAM services, at least 80 percent reported having a credentialing board or committee for acupuncture, chiropractic, and diet therapy. At least 80 percent of MTFs also reported having some form of review and approval process for acupressure, biofeedback, guided imagery, and progressive muscle relaxation. At least 20 percent of MTFs reported not having an established credentialing and privileging process for mindfulness meditation and stress management/relaxation therapy.

Detailed data on the entities charged with this responsibility for each CAM service, and for each of the combinations of CAM services defined by MTFs, are presented in Appendix H, Table H.15.

We also asked about the criteria used in the credentialing and privileging process for providers of CAM services in MTFs in which there was an established process. Respondents could select multiple criteria. One-half to two-thirds of CAM services across MTFs used certification, licensure, demonstrated performance, and special training as criteria for credentialing and privileging providers delivering CAM. Detailed data on provider criteria for each CAM service are presented in Appendix H, Table H.16.

Figure 6.4
Entities Responsible for Reviewing and Approving Credentials and Clinical Privileges for Providers Delivering the CAM Services Most Commonly Offered at MTFs

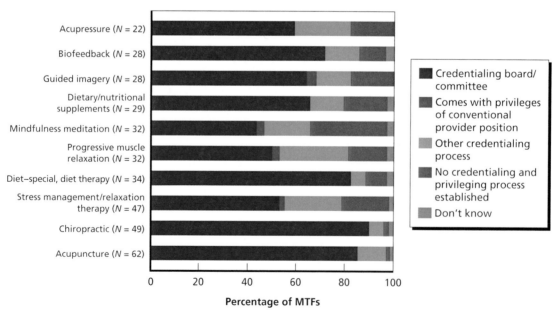

Training of New CAM Providers

MTFs that offer CAM were asked about the types of training for their new CAM providers (see Figure 6.5). Almost all MTFs (78 percent) offered training in using the electronic medical record (EMR) system (Armed Forces Health Longitudinal Technological Application [AHLTA]). About two-thirds of new CAM providers received training in medical charting and coding; 40 percent received training on the military health system structure and on how to make internal referrals. Several MTFs noted that they did not provide special training for CAM providers because their already-trained conventional practitioners were providing CAM.

Figure 6.5
Types of Training Given to CAM Providers When They Start Working in MTFs (*N* = 110)

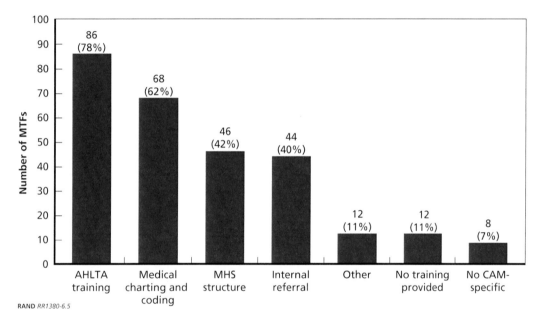

RAND *RR1380-6.5*

Practitioners Who Provide CAM at MTFs: Key Points

- According to the CAM survey, physicians (MDs/DOs), clinical psychologists, and licensed social workers are responsible for more than half of the estimated total 1,555 FTEs of MTF staff time devoted to CAM.
- Using the MHS utilization data, we estimate that chiropractors provide almost 70 percent of CAM visits for acupuncture, biofeedback, chiropractic, hypnosis/hypnotherapy, and massage. Different data collection methods are one explanation for this difference.
- Most CAM services are offered in outpatient settings, primarily in outpatient primary care and behavioral health, less frequently in outpatient pain clinics.
- About one-third of MTFs report that they offer at least some of their CAM services in an integrative health/medicine clinic or a CAM specialty clinic. CAM specialty clinics are slightly less common in smaller MTFs.
- Fifty percent to 60 percent of MTFs report open discussion of mutual patients and mutual referrals between CAM and conventional providers.
- Almost all MTFs report that primary care is a top referral source for patients interested in CAM, followed closely by referrals from various behavioral health providers. Two-thirds of MTFs also report self-/family or friend referral as a common source.
- The total MHS labor investment in CAM for 2015 is approximately $112.7 million. Most of this is MTF staff rather than contractor time.
- Most MTFs have a credentialing board or committee for providers, or another review and privileging process, for commonly offered CAM services.
- About two-thirds of MTFs cite certification, licensure, demonstrated performance, and special training as criteria for credentialing and privileging CAM providers.
- Most MTFs offer CAM providers training in the EMR system (AHLTA), and medical charting and coding.

CHAPTER SEVEN

CAM Coding and Documentation

We assessed the consistency with which each CAM service is documented in the EMR, including the availability and description of CPT procedure codes to document each CAM service, in the CAM survey. We also asked about the frequency of code use to document the treatment and inquired about how CAM services are documented in the EMR when CPT codes are not available.

At least half of MTFs report that commonly offered CAM services are "consistently documented in the electronic medical record (EMR), Armed Forces Health Longitudinal Technology Application (AHLTA)" with at least 90 percent of MTFs reporting consistently documenting chiropractic and acupuncture (Figure 7.1). However, up to one-third of MTFs were uncertain about the consistency of documentation for many common CAM services. In addition, documentation is not as consistent for less commonly offered CAM services, such as traditional Chinese medicine and animal-assisted therapy (see Appendix H, Table H.17).

The reported use of CPT codes to document common CAM services in the EMR was less common (Figure 7.2). At least 60 percent of MTFs reported that no CPT code existed for six of the ten most commonly offered CAM services. Only for chiropractic and acupuncture

Figure 7.1
MTFs That Reported Consistent Documentation of Common CAM Services in the EMR

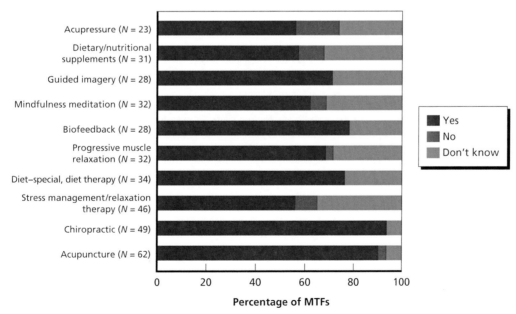

services did at least 50 percent of MTFs report using CPT codes to document every episode. When MTFs reported that CPT codes existed for CAM services, they were asked to supply the codes. Table 7.1 presents the CPT codes various MTFs reported using to document the utilization of the different types of CAM. Very few MTFs reported using other types of (non-CPT) codes to document CAM services. Therefore, Table 7.1 reports only CPT codes. The CPT codes reported suggest that some MTFs may use related or generic CPT codes when one does not exist for the specific CAM service. Detailed data on documentation and coding for specific CAM services are presented in Appendix H, Tables H.17 and H.18. Many CAM services do not have CPT codes available (Figure 7.2), and MTFs reported that CAM services are fairly consistently documented in the EMR (Figure 7.1)—these two facts suggest (and an MTF report confirms) that many procedures are documented only in text in the narrative section of the medical record.

Figure 7.2
CPT Procedure Codes Used to Document Common CAM Services in MTFs

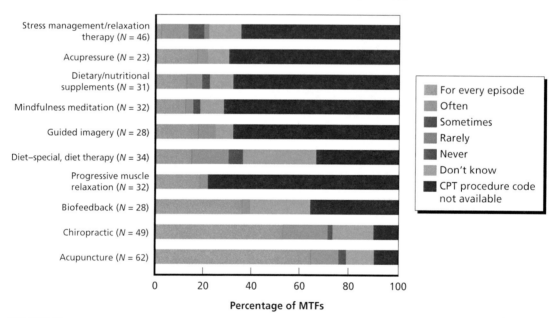

Table 7.1
CAM Activities Captured in CPT Codes

CAM Domain	CAM Activity	CPT Codes and Summary of Activity
Mind-body medicine	Animal-assisted therapy	• 97530 Therapeutic activities • 97532 Development of cognitive skills
	Biofeedback[a, b, c, d, g]	• 90901 Biofeedback • 97032 Alpha stimulation
	Guided imagery[a, b, e]	• 97530 Therapeutic activities • 97532 Development of cognitive skills • 90880 Hypnotherapy • 90901 Biofeedback
	Hypnosis/hypnotherapy [a]	• 90880 Hypnotherapy
	Meditation (includes all subgroups)[a, b, d, e, h]	
	Music therapy	• 97537 Sensory Integration
	Progressive muscle relaxation[a, b, c, e]	• 90901 Biofeedback
	Stress management, relaxation therapy [a,b,e,h]	• 90901 Biofeedback
	Yoga[c, g, h]	• 97530 Therapeutic activities • 97112 Neuromuscular reeducation
Biologically based practices	Diet–special, diet therapy[b, c]	• 97802–97804 Medical nutrition therapy
	Dietary/nutritional supplements	• 97802–97804 Medical nutrition therapy
Manipulative and body-based practices	Acupressure[f]	• 97810–97813 Acupuncture • 97140 Manual therapy techniques
	Acupuncture[e,f,h,j]	• 97810–97814 Acupuncture • 97140 Manual therapy techniques • 64550 TENS therapy • 97014, 97032 Electrical stimulation • 97141 Manipulation by physician
	Massage therapy[g]	• 97124 Massage • 97140 Manual therapy techniques • 97001, 97002 Physical therapy evaluation and reevaluation
	Movement practices (e.g., Feldenkreis, Pilates)[g, h]	• 97112 Neuromuscular reeducation • 97530 Therapeutic activities • 97150 Therapeutic procedure(s) for a group
	Chiropractic[f,g,h,i]	• 98941–98943 Chiropractic manipulation • 97140 Manual therapy techniques • 97112 Neuromuscular reeducation • 97810–97814 Acupuncture • 97530 Therapeutic activities • 99201–99215 Generic office visit • 73510 Diagnostic imaging
	Hyperbaric oxygen therapy	• 99183 Hyperbaric oxygen therapy • 97597, 97598, 97606 Wound debridement and wound management • 29581 Application of compression system

Table 7.1—Continued

CAM Domain	CAM Activity	CPT Codes and Summary of Activity
Energy Therapy	Tai chi, qi gong[c, g]	
Alternative or whole medical systems	Traditional Chinese medicine	• 97810–97814 Acupuncture

NOTE: Additional CPT codes used include the following:
[a] 90834, 90837: Psychotherapy, 45 or 60 minutes with patient and/or family member
[b] 96152, 96153: Health and behavior intervention, each 15 minutes, face-to-face; individual or group
[c] 96150: Health and behavior assessment, each 15 minutes, face-to-face
[d] 90875, 90876: Individual psychophysiological therapy incorporating biofeedback
[e] 90853: Group psychotherapy
[f] 98925-98929: Osteopathic manipulation
[g] 97110: Therapeutic exercises
[h] 97535, 98960: Self care/home-management training
[i] 97010, 97012, 97014, 97032: Applied modalities (electrical stimulation, hot/cold packs, and traction)
[j] 97026, 97028, 97035, 97039: Applied therapy (cold laser, ultraviolet, and infrared)

CAM Coding and Documentation: Key Points

- The majority of MTFs report that the use of commonly offered CAM services is "consistently documented in the electronic medical record."
- However, this documentation is often confined to a text-only entry because many MTFs report that the majority of commonly offered CAM services do not have an available CPT code.
- When CPT codes exist, MTFs report that they are usually used for documentation, particularly for chiropractic and acupuncture.
- Although the CAM-specific CPT codes are most commonly used when they exist, MTFs use a variety of other codes to document use of each type of CAM service.

CHAPTER EIGHT

Summary and Recommendations

This report provides the first systemwide look at the CAM services offered in the MHS. CAM services are widespread: 83 percent of MTFs offer one or more of a variety of CAM services for a variety of conditions, many of which can be difficult to treat with conventional medicine—e.g., chronic pain, stress, anxiety, and sleep disturbance. CAM services make up a substantial portion of the MHS: roughly 76,000 patient visits per month with 1,750 FTEs of staff and contractor time involved in delivering these services annually, and a minimum labor investment of $112.7 million per year. Patient visits for CAM make up a small but nontrivial portion of total outpatient MTF visits (approximately 7 percent).

However, there are barriers to the provision of CAM in the MTFs. MTFs cite not having the necessary providers as the most common reason for not offering CAM. Furthermore, while at least 80 percent of MTFs report having a credentialing board, committee, or other form of review process for most of the commonly offered types of CAM (to ensure only qualified providers deliver these therapies), at least 20 percent of MTFs report not having an established process for some CAM services, such as mindfulness meditation and stress management/relaxation therapy. There is also some inconsistency in the criteria used for credentialing and privileging. Standardization of credentialing and privileging would ensure that the practitioners who provide CAM services are properly trained.

There is also a need for better documentation and coding of the use of CAM services. Most MTFs reported that the use of the CAM services was consistently documented in the EMR. However, it is unclear how this could happen, because half of the services were reported as not having a CPT code, and others were reported documented with various CPT codes. For CAM services without a CPT code, information about their use would appear only in the narrative of a medical chart. Improved documentation and coding would facilitate better tracking of manpower use and needs, better record for physicians the other treatments that patients are receiving, and allow future studies focused on the safety, quality, and consistency of CAM services.

In general, our study's findings about CAM in MTFs are quite similar to results of the VA's CAM survey conducted in 2011 (Healthcare Analysis & Information Group, 2011). Similarities include the percentage of facilities offering CAM, the number of CAM types offered, reasons for offering and not offering CAM, the main conditions for which these treatments are used, the types of practitioners providing CAM, the credentialing and privileging of these providers and the criteria used, the evidence used to decide the offer of CAM services, the general number of estimated patient encounters per month, and how CAM services are documented and coded in the medical record. One important difference: VA did not include chiropractic in its survey because it is now considered mainstream, and no longer CAM, in the VHA.

There are, of course, differences between the studies. VA tends to have more facilities that offer, and more estimated patient encounters for, animal-assisted therapy, biofeedback, and music therapy, and fewer facilities that offer acupuncture (although the estimated number of patient encounters is similar) than the MHS. Probably because of this, the provider mix is also different. For example, physicians in the VA provide far fewer CAM services than are reported in MTFs.

As we discussed in Chapter Two, we are aware of the limitations inherent in our two data sources. Individuals assigned to this task at each MTF collected the CAM survey data. Respondents reported that they obtained the requested information by talking to individual CAM providers, staff in behavioral/mental health and primary care, and other health care providers. In MTFs that offer just a small number of CAM services, it is likely that a single individual or small group of people have adequate knowledge to accurately answer the survey. However, larger MTFs with numerous clinics may provide CAM services of which the MTF respondent was unaware, or a small group of people may not have sufficiently comprehensive knowledge of the CAM services provided to accurately answer all the questions in the CAM survey. We are grateful for their efforts but hope that this report will highlight the need for more formal and consistent systemwide data collection.

The health care utilization data that we used to supplement the CAM survey also have limitations. Specific procedure codes are available only for five general types of CAM: acupuncture, biofeedback, chiropractic, hypnosis/hypnotherapy, and massage therapy. Therefore, analyses based on the MHS data could address only these five therapies. The CAM survey results suggested some confusion on the availability of codes and how best to record the provision of CAM services in utilization data that would affect estimates of CAM use. First, multiple MTFs reported a lack of CPT codes for CAM, such as acupuncture, when such codes do exist, which would lead to an underestimate of CAM services used. For CAM without existing codes, some MTFs reported using related codes (e.g., using acupuncture codes for the provision of acupressure), which would lead to an overestimate of some CAM services, or the use of generic visit codes, which would lead to the use of CAM services not being identified in our analyses. The net effect of these conflicting inconsistencies is unknown.

However, despite the limitations in our data sources, we believe our comprehensive assessment of CAM services in the MHS makes an important contribution to ongoing efforts to understand the role of CAM in this context in order to better inform policies related to its provision and use. To further the goal of understanding the role of CAM in the MHS, we offer the following recommendations:

- **Standardize coding for CAM services.** The types of data sources the MTFs relied on for this study (e.g., mostly interviews with providers), and the data provided on coding and documentation underscore the need for more systematic data collection. Consistent tracking of the types of CAM services being offered, by what type of CAM provider and for which condition, will allow better management of manpower use and needs, a better record for physicians about the other treatments that patients are receiving, and easier data collection for future comparison studies. In particular:
  - Standardized coding should be developed for CAM services without a current specific CPT code.

- Because a number of CAM services are offered in combination (by the same provider for the same conditions and often in the same session), a standard way of coding should be developed for a predefined set of these combinations.

- **Conduct a medical record review at a small number of MTFs to validate survey findings and MHS utilization data.** Because MTFs report that almost all CAM use is consistently documented in the EMR, these records could be used to validate the data collected through the CAM survey, particularly the types of CAM offered, conditions for which CAM is used, the providers who are delivering these therapies and the time devoted to the provision, and patient encounters per month. Furthermore, given the reported inconsistency in the use of procedure codes to record CAM, a medical record review could also validate MHS utilization data for CAM in the selected MTFs, and could guide the standardization of CAM coding. Finally, the results of the validation study could inform whether additional audits of the MHS utilization data are needed for CAM services and how they should be targeted.

- **Address CAM in clinical guidelines for conditions for which it is frequently used.** More than half, but not all, of MTFs cited scientific evidence as a reason to offer their CAM therapies. Addressing CAM in the clinical guidelines will facilitate providers having access to the scientific evidence on the safety, efficacy, and effectiveness of CAM therapies for specific conditions and should help support better-informed decisions by MTF commanders, clinical leaders, and individual providers about the types of CAM to offer and conditions these therapies are best used to treat. DCoE has initiated this process by funding a series of systematic reviews for selected CAM services and conditions, which have informed VA/DoD clinical guidelines. We encourage the continuation of this activity focusing on the high-frequency-condition/CAM combinations identified in this report.

- **Standardize credentialing and privileging.** A standardized protocol for credentialing and privileging the providers of CAM services should be developed to ensure that the providers are properly and consistently trained, and to assist MTFs in credentialing and privileging new CAM providers.

- **Conduct outcomes research.** Some CAM service/condition combinations were associated with reports of symptom improvement and/or medication reduction. Future outcomes research might appropriately target these services, especially if other MTFs are thinking of offering them and/or if sufficient relevant clinical studies do not already exist.

We believe implementation of these recommendations will improve patient care through the mechanisms outlined above and help assure the safety, quality, consistency, and appropriate availability of CAM services.

Acupuncture at a Glance

Definition

Acupuncture is the stimulation of specific points on the body through the insertion of thin metal needles through the skin.

Number of MTFs Offering Acupuncture

Acupuncture is offered at 76 MTFs. This is 57 percent of the 133 MTFs that responded to the CAM survey, and 69 percent of the 110 MTFs that offer CAM. An additional 20 MTFs recommend off-site acupuncture to their patients. It is the second most common CAM referral from conventional medicine, and a total of 105 MTFs (79 percent of 133) indicated that acupuncture was in the top three of CAM services they would be most interested in offering (including whether it is already offered at their MTF).

Acupuncture is sometimes used in combination with other CAM therapies. In five MTFs, it is offered in combination with other manipulative and body-based CAM therapies, such as acupressure and chiropractic. In 20 MTFs, it is offered in combination with a variety of other CAM services. For example, acupuncture could be offered as part of a mixed package of CAM services along with acupressure, chiropractic, progressive muscle relaxation, stress management/relaxation therapy, yoga, and biofeedback. Because the data for these combinations could not be separated by CAM therapy, the remainder of this appendix will include only data on the 62 MTFs that reported on acupuncture delivered on its own, separate from other types of CAM.

Conditions for Which Acupuncture Is Used

MTFs reported using acupuncture most often as a treatment for various types of pain: chronic pain (92 percent of MTFs offering acupuncture) and back pain (89 percent), followed closely by non–TBI-related headache (82 percent), acute pain (e.g., posttrauma/injury or preoperative or postoperative; 79 percent), arthritis (55 percent) and pain related to TBI (50 percent). Acupuncture is also commonly used in the treatment of psychological health conditions: anxiety disorder (52 percent), sleep disturbance (50 percent), stress management (48 percent), depression (45 percent), posttraumatic stress disorder and acute stress disorder (40 percent), tobacco dependence (39 percent), and other substance abuse disorders (29 percent). However, acupuncture seems to be used for almost all conditions. Three or more of the MTFs offering acupuncture endorsed each of the 24 conditions listed in the survey as a use.

Figure A.1, based on an analysis of 2013 MHS outpatient direct care utilization data, generally supports what was found in the CAM survey. Note that MHS data report on the number of times an acupuncture code was used (i.e., generally, numbers of visits) and the CAM survey reports results by number of MTFs. Nevertheless, in both cases acupuncture is used most often for pain.

It is believed that patients are highly adherent with acupuncture. More than half (56 percent) of MTFs report high patient adherence (i.e., patients attend 70 percent to 100 percent of prescribed sessions), another almost quarter (24 percent) report moderate adherence (i.e., that patients attend 30 percent to 70 percent of prescribed sessions), and 18 percent said that they did not know about patient adherence.

MTFs also reported that acupuncture is highly effective as measured by patient and provider report of success in symptom reductions and in observed reductions in medication use. Of the MTFs answering these questions, 92 percent reported that acupuncture shows the most success in reducing pain. Two-thirds (66 percent) said acupuncture improves patients' quality of life, 56 percent said it improves patient satisfaction, 53 percent said it improves sleep, and 50 percent reported that it reduces stress. One-quarter to one-half of MTFs reported success in reducing anxiety symptoms; improving functional status; improving work performance; improving self-management skills, self-regulation and awareness; reducing PTSD symptoms; increasing healthy behaviors; and reducing depressive symptoms. The majority (61 percent) of these MTFs also reported an observed reduction in medication use, while more than one-third (36 percent) said that they did not know whether medication use was reduced. The most frequently reported observed medication reduction was for analgesics (97 percent of MTFs that reported an observed medication reduction), followed by sleep medications (44 percent), anxiolytics (42 percent), and antidepressants (19 percent).

Figure A.1
Acupuncture Procedures in 2013 MHS Utilization Data

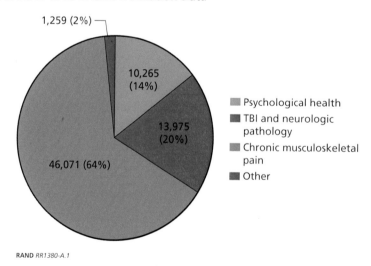

Patient Demand for Acupuncture

Acupuncture is the fifth most popular CAM service in terms of patient demand. Demand across all MTFs that offer acupuncture is estimated to be about 5,500 (3,000 to 8,000) patient encounters per month. It should be noted that an analysis of 2013 outpatient MHS utilization data showed an average of more than 3,700 visits for acupuncture per month, so the estimate from the CAM survey of MTFs of 5,500 may be a little high but is within the low-high estimate range. When asked whether there was a waiting list for acupuncture appointments, almost half (47 percent) of MTFs said there was, almost one-third (31 percent) said there wasn't and the others (23 percent) reported that they did not know. Of those reporting a wait list, almost a half said that it contained fewer than ten patients, but more than one-third had wait lists of 40 patients or more. The rest reported wait lists of ten to 40 patients.

Provider Characteristics

The MTFs report that a total of 216 FTEs of MTF staff time, plus about five FTEs of contractor and volunteer time, was spent over the year offering acupuncture. Physicians deliver the majority of acupuncture (MDs/DOs; 76 percent of the staff time devoted to acupuncture and 68 percent of contractor and volunteer time). The next most common providers of acupuncture are licensed acupuncturists (10 percent of staff time and 21 percent of contractor and volunteer time).

The fact that physicians provided most of the acupuncture services is confirmed by an analysis of 2013 MHS utilization data that shows more than half (52 percent) of the coded acupuncture visits that year were from physicians (MDs/DOs). Physical or occupational therapists (20 percent) were the next largest provider group using acupuncture codes in the MHS utilization data, followed by other (includes optometry, audiology, pharmacists, lab and pathology technicians, corpsmen, medical chemists, and students; 11 percent), chiropractors (8 percent) and behavioral health practitioners (6 percent). Some of the differences seen in what MTFs reported in the survey could have to do with the types of providers who are allowed to use CPT codes in the MHS system.

The individuals or groups with responsibility for reviewing and approving clinical privileges for providers delivering acupuncture include a credentialing board or committee in the vast majority of MTFs (85 percent). More than 40 percent of MTFs report approval responsibility lies (or also lies) with administration or leadership (e.g., the chief of medical staff), and/or almost 30 percent report that it lies with the provider's supervisor (29 percent). The following criteria were used during the credentialing and privileging process for providers delivering acupuncture: certification (90 percent), special training (69 percent), demonstrated performance (52 percent), and licensure (44 percent).

Coding and Documentation

CPT codes exist for acupuncture: 97810, 97811, 97813, and 97814 for 15-minute increments of acupuncture involving one or more needles, with or without electrical stimulation. While most MTFs reported they used these codes to document acupuncture in the EMR,

10 percent of MTFs report that a CPT code is not available for acupuncture. More than 90 percent of MTFs report that the provision of acupuncture is consistently documented in the EMR, and another 6 percent say that they do not know whether acupuncture is consistently documented in the EMR. Of those that noted CPT codes available for acupuncture, almost three-quarters (71 percent) report that every episode of acupuncture is documented using these CPT codes, another 13 percent say that episodes are often documented, and 13 percent say that they do not know how often codes are reported for acupuncture.

Chiropractic at a Glance

Definition

Chiropractic care focuses on the relationship between the body's structure—mainly the spine—and functioning. Although practitioners may use a variety of treatment approaches, they primarily perform adjustments (i.e., manipulations) to the spine or other parts of the body with the goal of correcting alignment problems, alleviating pain, improving function, and supporting the body's natural ability to heal itself.

Number of MTFs Offering Chiropractic

Chiropractic is offered at 60 MTFs. This is 45 percent of the 133 MTFs that responded to the CAM survey, and 55 percent of the 110 MTFs that offer CAM. An additional 32 MTFs recommend off-site chiropractic to their patients. It is the third most common CAM referral from conventional medicine, and a total of 84 MTFs (63 percent of 133) indicated that chiropractic was in the top three of CAM services they would be most interested in offering (including whether it is already offered at their MTF).

Chiropractic is sometimes used in combination with other CAM therapies. In two MTFs, it is offered in combination with other manipulative and body-based CAM therapies, such as acupuncture and massage. In 12 MTFs, it is offered in combination with a variety of other CAM services. For example, chiropractic could be offered as part of a package of CAM services along with acupuncture, acupressure, progressive muscle relaxation, stress management/relaxation therapy, yoga, and biofeedback. Because the data for these combinations could not be separated by CAM therapy, the remainder of this appendix will include only data on the 49 MTFs that reported on chiropractic delivered on its own, separate from other types of CAM.

Conditions for Which Chiropractic Is Used

MTFs reported using chiropractic almost exclusively to treat various types of pain: back pain (96 percent of MTFs offering chiropractic) and chronic pain (90 percent), followed closely by non-TBI-related headache (61 percent), acute pain (e.g., posttrauma/injury or preoperative or postoperative; 61 percent), arthritis (51 percent), and pain related to TBI (41 percent). The only other uses endorsed by 10 percent or more MTFs are improving general health, wellness and prevention (24 percent), and resilience promotion (16 percent).

Figure B.1, based on an analysis of 2013 MHS outpatient data, generally supports what was found in the CAM survey. Note that MHS data report on the number of times a chiropractic code was used (i.e., roughly the number of visits), and the CAM survey reports results by number of MTFs. Nevertheless, in both cases chiropractic care is used almost exclusively for pain.

It is believed that patients are highly adherent with chiropractic. More than 60 percent of MTFs report high patient adherence (i.e., patients attend 70 percent to 100 percent of prescribed sessions), 22 percent report moderate adherence (i.e., patients attend 30 percent to 70 percent of prescribed sessions), and 16 percent report that they did not know about patient adherence for chiropractic.

MTFs also reported that chiropractic is highly effective as measured by patient and provider report of success in symptom reductions and in observed reductions in medications of different types. Of the MTFs answering these questions, 94 percent reported that chiropractic shows the most success in reducing pain. Almost two-thirds (65 percent and 63 percent) said chiropractic improves patient satisfaction and patients' quality of life, 57 percent reported it improves functional status, 55 percent said it improves work performance, and 45 percent said it improves sleep. About one-quarter to 30 percent of MTFs reported increased healthy behaviors, increased military retention, reduced stress, and improved self-management skills, self-regulation and awareness. The majority (59 percent) of these MTFs also reported an observed reduction in medication use with chiropractic, while more than one-third (39 percent) said that they did not know whether medication use was reduced. All (100 percent) of MTFs that reported an observed medication reduction reported a reduction in analgesics. Twenty-two percent reported a reduction in sleep medications; a few MTFs reported reduced use of both anxiolytics and antidepressants (7 percent each).

Figure B.1
Chiropractic Procedures in 2013 MHS Utilization Data

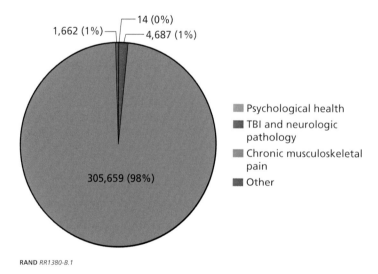

Patient Demand for Chiropractic

Chiropractic is the most popular CAM service in terms of patient demand. Demand across all MTFs that offer chiropractic separate from other CAM services is estimated to be 14,000 (9,250 to 18,750) patient encounters per month. It should be noted that an analysis of 2013 outpatient MHS data showed an average of 25,000 visits coded for chiropractic manipulation per month, so the estimate from the CAM survey of 14,000 may be too low, even if the chiropractic-related portion of the 11,350 patient encounters for mixed combinations of CAM is considered. When asked whether there was a waiting list for chiropractic appointments, 43 percent of MTFs said there was a list, more than one-quarter (27 percent) said there wasn't, and the others (31 percent) reported that they did not know of a waiting list. Of those reporting a wait list, almost a half said that it contained more than 40 patients, and almost 20 percent had wait lists of fewer than 10 patients. The rest reported wait lists of ten to 40 patients.

Provider Characteristics

The MTFs report that a total of 54 FTEs of MTF staff time, plus about 18 FTEs of contractor and volunteer time was spent over the year offering chiropractic care. Not surprisingly, the vast majority of chiropractic care is being delivered by chiropractors (83 percent of the staff time devoted to chiropractic and 94 percent of contractor and volunteer time). The next most common providers of chiropractic care are physicians (MDs/DOs)—8 percent of staff time—and physical or occupational therapists—5 percent of staff time.

An analysis of 2013 MHS utilization data shows that almost all (97 percent) the visits coded for chiropractic manipulation that year were provided by chiropractors, which is consistent with what was reported by the MTFs.

The individuals or groups with responsibility for reviewing and approving clinical privileges for providers delivering chiropractic care include a credentialing board or committee in the vast majority of MTFs (90 percent). Almost 40 percent of MTFs report approval responsibility lies (or also lies) with administration or leadership (e.g., the chief of medical staff), and almost 30 percent report that it lies with the provider's supervisor. The following criteria were used during the credentialing and privileging process for providers delivering acupuncture: licensure (83 percent), certification (79 percent), demonstrated performance (60 percent), and special training (52 percent).

Coding and Documentation

CPT codes exist for chiropractic: 98940, 98941, 98942, and 98943 for chiropractic manipulative therapy to different body regions and numbers of regions. However, four to five MTFs each also reported the use of the following codes for chiropractic: osteopathic manipulation (98925 to 98929), manual therapy techniques (97140), acupuncture (97810 to 97814), and general office visits (99201 to 99215). Nevertheless, 10 percent of MTFs incorrectly report that a CPT code is not available for chiropractic. More than 90 percent (94 percent) of MTFs report that the provision of chiropractic care is consistently documented in the EMR, and the remaining 6 percent of MTFs say that they do not know whether chiropractic care is consistently documented in EMRs. Of those that reported CPT codes available for chiropractic, about 60 percent (59 percent) report that every episode of chiropractic care is documented using the CPT codes listed, another 20 percent say that it is often documented, and 18 percent say they do not know how often chiropractic care is documented using CPT codes.

Diet Therapy at a Glance

Definition

Major dietary changes to promote health not related to allergies or intolerance and not part of the U.S. Department of Agriculture's dietary guidelines (e.g., blood type diet, raw food diet, etc.), which may include significant reductions or increases in certain daily nutrient intake requirements.

Number of MTFs Offering Diet Therapy

Diet therapy is offered at 52 MTFs. This is 39 percent of the 133 MTFs that responded to the survey, and 47 percent of the 110 MTFs that offer CAM. An additional 20 MTFs recommend off-site diet therapy to their patients. It is the fourth most common CAM referral from conventional medicine, and a total of 29 MTFs (22 percent of 133) indicated that diet therapy was in the top three of CAM services they would be most interested in offering (including whether it is already offered at their MTF).

Diet therapy is sometimes used in combination with other CAM therapies. For example, ten MTFs report its use in combination with nutritional supplements, and, in two cases, also with herbs. Because these combinations (called biologically based combinations) are reasonably close to diet therapy itself, the results of this combination will be included with data from the 34 MTFs that reported on diet therapy use alone (for a total of 44 MTF reports) in the remainder of this appendix. Fifteen MTFs reported on diet therapy use combined with a number of different types of CAM. For example, diet therapy could be offered as part of a mixed package of CAM services along with acupuncture, stress management/relaxation therapy, yoga, guided imagery, massage therapy, chiropractic, movement practices, and biofeedback. Because the data for these mixed combinations could not be separated by CAM therapy, the remainder of this appendix will include only data on the 34 MTFs that reported on diet therapy delivered on its own, separate from other types of CAM, and on the ten MTFs that reported on biologically based combinations, for a total of 44 MTFs.

Conditions for Which Diet Therapy Is Used

MTFs reported using diet therapy most often for various types of chronic disease: mainly obesity (80 percent of MTFs), diabetes (77 percent), heart disease (73 percent), and hypertension (70 percent). It is also commonly used for weight loss (70 percent) and general health, wellness, and prevention (61 percent). Twenty percent to 30 percent of MTFs also report using diet therapy for resilience promotion (27 percent), cancer (25 percent), chronic pain (23 percent), and non-TBI-related headache (20 percent).

It is believed that patients are moderately adherent with this therapy. Thirty-five percent of MTFs report moderate patient adherence (i.e., patients attend 30 percent to 70 percent of prescribed sessions), and 14 percent each report high adherence (i.e., patients attend 70 percent to 100 percent of prescribed sessions) and low adherence (i.e., patients attend less than 30 percent of prescribed sessions). Thirty percent of MTFs reported that they did not know about patient adherence to diet therapies.

MTFs reported that diet therapy shows the most success as measured by patient and provider report: increasing healthy behaviors (66 percent); and improving quality of life (57 percent), functional health status (45 percent), patient satisfaction (43 percent), work performance (30 percent), and self-management skills, self-regulation and awareness (27 percent). Only one or two MTFs each reported an observed reduction in analgesics, antidepressants, anxiolytics, and sleep medications associated with the use of diet therapy.

Patient Demand for Diet Therapy

Diet therapy is the fourth most popular CAM service in terms of patient demand. Demand across all MTFs that offer diet therapy is estimated to be almost 6,000 (3,800 to 8,100) patient encounters per month. Because this therapy does not have specific CPT codes, it was not addressed in the MHS utilization data analysis. When asked whether there was a waiting list for diet therapy appointments, about 20 percent of MTFs said there was, more than one-third (34 percent) said there wasn't, and the others (45 percent) reported that they did not know about wait lists. Of those reporting a wait list, two-thirds said that it contained fewer than ten patients, and none reported wait lists of more than 40 patients. The rest reported wait lists of ten to 40 patients.

Provider Characteristics

The MTFs report that a total of 98 FTEs of MTF staff time, plus 15 FTEs of contractor and volunteer time, were spent over the year offering diet therapy. Not surprisingly, dietitians deliver the largest proportion of diet therapy (33 percent of the staff time devoted to diet therapy and 54 percent of contractor and volunteer time). The next most common MTF staff providers of diet therapy are physicians (MDs/DOs; 15 percent of staff FTEs) and registered nurses (11 percent). The next most common contractor or volunteer providers of diet therapy are chiropractors (13 percent of contractor or volunteer FTEs), and CAM-specific providers (trained and/or licensed in a specific modality; 13 percent).

The individuals or groups with responsibility for reviewing and approving clinical privileges for providers delivering diet therapy include a credentialing board or committee in the vast majority of MTFs (80 percent). One-third of MTFs report approval responsibility lies (or also lies) with administration or leadership (e.g., the chief of medical staff), and/or 16 percent report that it lies with the provider's supervisor. The following criteria were used during the credentialing and privileging process for providers delivering diet therapy: certification (73 percent), licensure (70 percent), demonstrated performance (40 percent), and special training (28 percent).

Coding and Documentation

MTFs reported that diet therapy is usually coded using the set of CPT codes for medical nutrition therapy: 97802 to 97804 for initial visits, follow-up visits, and group visits, respectively. However, one-third of MTFs report that a CPT procedure code is not available for diet therapy. Almost 80 percent of MTFs report that the provision of diet therapy is consistently documented in the EMR, and the remaining MTFs say that they do not know about document of diet therapy in EMRs. Of those that reported CPT codes available for diet therapy, 21 percent report that every episode of diet therapy is documented using these CPT codes, another 21 percent say that it is often documented, and 43 percent say that they do not know about frequency of CPT code use for diet therapy.

Mindfulness Meditation at a Glance

Definition

Mindfulness meditation is form of meditation where the focus of attention is on a physical sensation, such as breathing, with the intent to increase awareness of the present.

Number of MTFs Offering Mindfulness Meditation

Mindfulness meditation is offered at 56 MTFs. This is 42 percent of the 133 MTFs that responded to the survey, and 51 percent of the 110 MTFs that offer CAM. An additional 17 MTFs recommend off-site mindfulness meditation to their patients. It is the sixth most common CAM referral from conventional medicine, and a total of 16 MTFs (12 percent of 133) indicated that mindfulness meditation was in the top three of CAM services they would be most interested in offering (including whether it is already offered at their MTF).

Mindfulness meditation is sometimes used in combination with other CAM therapies. Thirty MTFs reported using mindfulness meditation in combination with other mind-body therapies, such as progressive muscle relaxation and stress management/relaxation therapy. Mindfulness meditation was used in combination with a broader set of other CAM services by 19 MTFs. For example, mindfulness meditation could be offered as part of a mixed package of CAM services along with acupuncture, acupressure, stress management/relaxation therapy, diet therapy, nutritional supplements, yoga, aromatherapy, massage therapy, chiropractic, and progressive muscle relaxation. Because the data on these combinations could not be separated by CAM therapy, the remainder of this appendix will report only on the responses of the 32 MTFs that reported on mindfulness meditation alone. Appendix E reports on the mind-body combinations separate from stress management/relaxation therapy.

Conditions for Which Mindfulness Meditation Is Used

MTFs reported using mindfulness meditation most often to improve psychological health: anxiety disorder (91 percent of MTFs offering mindfulness meditation), stress management (88 percent), depression (88 percent), posttraumatic stress disorder and acute stress disorder (78 percent), sleep disturbance (75 percent), and other substance abuse disorders (53 percent).

It is also often used for general health, wellness and prevention (59 percent), chronic pain (53 percent), and resilience promotion (50 percent). Twenty percent to 35 percent of MTFs also report using mindfulness meditation for: back pain, neurological symptoms related to TBI, non-TBI-related headaches, acute pain, tobacco dependence, hypertension, arthritis, weight loss, and obesity.

MTFs report that patients are moderately adherent with mindfulness meditation. Thirty-eight percent of MTFs that answered this question report moderate patient adherence (i.e., patients attend 30 percent to 70 percent of prescribed sessions). Another 25 percent report high adherence (i.e., that patients attend 70 percent to 100 percent of prescribed sessions) and less than 10 percent report low adherence (i.e., patients attend less than 30 percent of prescribed sessions). The remaining MTFs (28 percent) report that they don't know the patient adherence for mindfulness meditation.

MTFs also reported that mindfulness meditation is highly effective as measured by patient and provider report of success in symptom reductions and in observed reductions in medications of different types. Of the MTFs answering these questions, 88 percent reported that mindfulness meditation shows the most success in reducing anxiety symptoms, followed closely by 84 percent reporting that it showed success in reducing stress. The therapy was also reported as having success in improving quality of life (63 percent); improving sleep (59 percent); improving self-management skills, self-regulation, and awareness (56 percent); reducing PTSD symptoms (53 percent); reducing depression (47 percent); increasing healthy behaviors (44 percent); improving patient satisfaction (41 percent); improving work performance (41 percent); and reducing pain (34 percent). One-third (34 percent) of these MTFs also reported an observed reduction in medication use associated with mindfulness meditation, while about half (52 percent) said that they did not know whether medication use was reduced as a result of this therapy. The highest report of observed reductions in medication use was for analgesics and anxiolytics (70 percent of MTFs that reported an observed medication reduction), followed by sleep medications (60 percent).

Patient Demand for Mindfulness Meditation

Mindfulness meditation, when considered by itself, is the ninth most popular CAM service in terms of patient demand. Demand across all MTFs that reported on mindfulness meditation alone is estimated to be 2,500 (1,450 to 3,550) patient encounters per month. Because this therapy does not have specific CPT codes, it was not addressed in the MHS utilization data analysis. When asked whether there was a wait list for mindfulness meditation, a quarter (25 percent) of MTFs said there was, 59 percent said there was not, and the others (16 percent) reported that they did not know whether there was a wait list. Of those reporting a wait list, half said that it contained fewer than ten patients, and a quarter reported wait lists of more than 40 patients. The rest reported wait lists of ten to 40 patients.

Provider Characteristics

The MTFs report that a total of 58 FTEs of MTF staff time, plus about 4.5 FTEs of contractor and volunteer time, was spent over the year offering mindfulness meditation. Clinical psychologists are the largest group in both categories (46 percent of the staff time devoted to mindfulness meditation and 53 percent of contractor and volunteer time). The bulk of the remainder of staff time is provided by social workers (27 percent). The remainder of the contractor and volunteer time comes from professional licensed counselors (23 percent) and physical therapy/occupational therapy technicians (23 percent).

The individuals or groups with responsibility for reviewing and approving clinical privileges for providers delivering mindfulness meditation includes a credentialing board or committee (44 percent), administration or leadership (e.g., the chief of medical staff; 31 percent), and the provider's supervisor (22 percent). Another 31 percent of MTFs report that no credentialing and privileging process has been established. For those MTFs reporting a process, the following criteria were used during the credentialing and privileging process for providers delivering mindfulness meditation: licensure (64 percent), special training (55 percent), demonstrated performance (50 percent), and certification (41 percent).

Coding and Documentation

Almost three-quarters (72 percent) of MTFs report that a CPT code is not available for mindfulness meditation. Of the MTFs reporting codes, the only ones reported by more than one MTF were 90834 and 90837 (psychotherapy for 45 or 60 minutes with a patient and/or family member). Almost two-thirds (63 percent) of MTFs report that the provision of mindfulness meditation is consistently documented in the EMR, and another 31 percent say that they do not know whether it is consistently documented. Of those that reported using CPT codes for mindfulness meditation, less than half (44 percent) report that every episode of mindfulness meditation is documented using the reported CPT codes.

Stress Management/Relaxation Therapy at a Glance

Definition

Relaxation therapy is a broad term used to describe a number of techniques that promote stress reduction, the elimination of tension throughout the body, and a calm and peaceful state of mind.

Number of MTFs Offering Stress Management/Relaxation Therapy

Relaxation therapy is offered at 83 MTFs. This is 62 percent of the 133 MTFs that responded to the CAM survey, and 75 percent of the 110 MTFs that offer CAM. An additional 12 MTFs recommend off-site relaxation therapy to their patients. It is the most common CAM referral from conventional medicine, and a total of 30 MTFs (23 percent of 133) indicated that relaxation therapy was in the top three of CAM services they would be most interested in offering (including whether it is already offered at their MTF).

Relaxation therapy is often used in combination with other CAM therapies. Forty-two MTFs reported using stress management/relaxation therapy in combination with other mind-body therapies, such as progressive muscle relaxation and mindfulness meditation. Because these mind-body combinations are reasonably close to relaxation therapy itself, the results of these combinations, for the 44 MTFs that offer them, will be reported alongside data from the 46 MTFs that reported on relaxation therapy use alone in the remainder of this appendix. Twenty-six MTFs reported using relaxation therapy in combination with a number of different types of CAM; for example, relaxation therapy could be offered as part of a mixed package of CAM services along with acupuncture, acupressure, mindfulness meditation, diet therapy, nutritional supplements, yoga, aromatherapy, massage therapy, chiropractic, and progressive muscle relaxation. Because of the variety of CAM therapies involved and the fact that these data could not be separated by CAM therapy, these mixed combinations will not be included in the remainder of this appendix.

Conditions for Which Relaxation Therapy Is Used

Not surprisingly, MTFs most often reported using relaxation therapy for stress management (98 percent of MTFs answering this question for relaxation therapy), followed closely by treatment for anxiety (89 percent). Relaxation therapy is also commonly used in the treatment of sleep disturbance, PTSD and acute stress disorder, and depression by more than two-thirds of MTFs each (70 percent, 70 percent, and 67 percent, respectively). One-quarter to one-half of MTFs also report the use of relaxation therapy for chronic pain; substance use disorder; general health, wellness and prevention; resilience promotion; back pain; non-TBI-related headache; pain related to TBI; and acute pain.

MTFs most often report mind-body combinations for treatment of anxiety (98 percent of MTFs reporting on one or more of these combinations), stress management (93 percent), PTSD and acute stress disorder (91 percent), and depression (91 percent). These are followed closely by treatment use for general health, wellness, and prevention (68 percent), chronic pain (64 percent), nontobacco substance use disorder (55 percent), non-TBI-related headache (52 percent), and resilience promotion (52 percent). One-quarter to one-half of MTFs also report the use of mind-body combinations for tobacco dependence, back pain, pain related to TBI, weight loss, neurological symptoms related to TBI, acute pain (posttrauma/injury, preoperative, postoperative), arthritis, obesity, and hypertension.

MTFs reported that patients are moderately adherent with relaxation therapy. One-third of MTFs report moderate patient adherence (i.e., patients attend 30 percent to 70 percent of prescribed sessions), almost 40 percent (39 percent) report that they don't know about patient adherence to relaxation therapy, and the remaining MTFs report high adherence (i.e., patients attend 70 percent to 100 percent of prescribed sessions). Patients are also reported to be moderately adherent with the mind-body combinations. About one-third of MTFs report moderate patient adherence (i.e., that patients attend 30 percent to 70 percent of prescribed sessions), 23 percent report that they don't know about adherence to mind-body combinations, and most of the remaining MTFs report high adherence (i.e., patients attend 70 percent to 100 percent of prescribed sessions).

MTFs reported that relaxation therapy is highly effective as measured by patient and provider report of success in reducing symptoms. Of the MTFs answering these questions, 87 percent reported that relaxation therapy shows the most success in reducing stress, followed closely by 80 percent reporting that it showed success in reducing anxiety. This therapy also seems to have some success in improving quality of life, sleep and self-management skills, self-regulation, and awareness, with about half of MTFs reporting success for each. One-third to one-half of MTFs also reported relaxation therapy reduced PTSD symptoms, depressive symptoms, and pain; improved work performance and patient satisfaction; and increased healthy behaviors.

MTFs also reported that mind-body CAM combinations are highly effective and may be slightly more effective than relaxation therapy alone as measured by patient and provider report of success in reducing symptoms. Of the MTFs answering these questions for the mind-body combinations, 91 percent reported that they show the most success in reducing anxiety, followed closely by 86 percent reporting that it showed success in reducing stress and 75 percent reporting improved quality of life. These combination therapies also seem to have some success in reducing depression, PTSD symptoms, and pain; improving functional health status, patient satisfaction, sleep, self-management skills, self-regulation, and awareness, and work performance; and increasing healthy behaviors, with about half to two-thirds of MTFs reporting each.

About one-fifth (21 percent) of MTFs reported an observed reduction in medication use associated with relaxation therapy, while almost two-thirds (64 percent) said that they do not know if medication use reductions occurred as a result of this therapy. All (100 percent) of the MTFs that reported an observed medication reduction reported reductions in anxiolytics.

More than one-third (37 percent) of MTFs reporting on mind-body combinations said that they observed a reduction in medication use associated with the use of these combinations, while almost half (49 percent) said that they did not know whether use of mind-body combinations was associated with a reduction in use of medication. Of those MTFs that reported a medication use reduction with mind-body combinations, 80 percent reported a reduction in sleep medications, 60 percent reported decreased use of analgesics, and roughly half reported a reduction in antidepressants and anxiolytics.

Patient Demand for Stress Management/Relaxation Therapy

Relaxation therapy is the sixth most popular CAM service in terms of patient demand when use is considered separate from other CAM therapies, and mind-body combinations are the third most popular CAM service. Demand across all MTFs that report offering relaxation therapy alone is estimated to be 4,300 (2,350 to 6,300) patient encounters per month, and demand for the mind-body combinations is estimated to be 8,500 (5,450 to 11,650) patient encounters per month. Because these therapies do not have specific CPT codes, they were not addressed in the MHS utilization data analysis.

When asked whether there was a waiting list for relaxation therapy, a quarter (26 percent) of MTFs said there was, more than one-half (57 percent) said there was not, and the others (17 percent) reported that they did not know whether there was a wait list for relaxation therapy. Of those reporting a wait list, almost 60 percent said that it contained fewer than ten patients, and a quarter reported wait lists of more than 40 patients. The rest reported wait lists of ten to 40 patients. Results were similar for the mind-body combinations. When asked whether there was a waiting list for the combination mind-body therapies, almost a quarter (23 percent) of MTFs said there was, more than one-half (57 percent) said there was not, and the others (20 percent) reported that they did not know whether there was a wait list for mind-body combinations. Of those reporting a wait list for mind-body combinations, 60 percent said that it contained fewer than ten patients, and 20 percent reported wait lists of more than 40 patients.

Provider Characteristics

The MTFs report that a total of 155 FTEs of MTF staff time, plus about 58 FTEs of contractor and volunteer time, was spent over the year offering relaxation therapy. Clinical psychologists are the largest group in both categories (42 percent of the staff time devoted to relaxation therapy and 19 percent of contractor and volunteer time). The bulk of the remainder of staff time is provided by social workers (28 percent). The remainder of the contractor and volunteer time comes from physicians (MDs/DOs; 14 percent), social workers (12 percent), and professional licensed counselors (10 percent).

The MTFs with mind-body combinations report fewer FTEs of staff (127 FTEs) and contractors or volunteers (17 FTEs) time than was seen for relaxation therapy. Again, clinical psychologists are the largest group in both categories (42 percent of the staff time devoted to mindfulness meditation and 67 percent of contractor and volunteer time). The bulk of the remainder of staff time is provided by social workers (32 percent). The remainder of the contractor and volunteer time mostly comes from professional licensed counselors (11 percent).

The main individuals or groups with responsibility for reviewing and approving clinical privileges for providers delivering relaxation therapy includes a credentialing board or committee (53 percent), administration or leadership (e.g., the chief of medical staff; 43 percent), and the provider's supervisor (26 percent). Nineteen percent of MTFs report that no credentialing and privileging process has been established. Of MTFs with a process in place, the following criteria were used during the credentialing and privileging process for providers delivering relaxation therapy: licensure (63 percent), demonstrated performance (58 percent), special training (47 percent), and certification (45 percent).

The credentialing and privileging situation is similar for providers of the mind-body combinations with the exception of a larger emphasis on certification. The main individuals or groups with responsibility for reviewing and approving clinical privileges for providers delivering the combination mind-body therapies include a credentialing board or committee (67 percent), administration or leadership (e.g., the chief of medical staff; 46 percent), and the provider's supervisor (35 percent). Sixteen percent of MTFs report that no credentialing and privileging process has been established. Of MTFs with a process in place, the following criteria were used during the credentialing and privileging process for providers delivering the combination mind-body therapies: certification (76 percent), licensure (73 percent), demonstrated performance (68 percent), and special training (54 percent).

Coding and Documentation

Almost two-thirds (63 percent) of MTFs report that there is no CPT procedure code available for relaxation therapy. Of the MTFs reporting codes, the only ones reported by more than one MTF were 90834 and 90837 (psychotherapy for 45 or 60 minutes with a patient and/or family member), 90901 (biofeedback), and 96152 (health and behavioral intervention, 15 minutes, for an individual). Data on the codes used are not available for the mind-body combinations. Even with the lack of CPT codes, 77 percent of MTFs reporting on these therapies said that their use is consistently documented in the EMR, and 14 percent said they did not know about the consistency of data code use. More than one-half (57 percent) of MTFs that reported on relaxation therapy alone said that the provision of relaxation therapy is consistently documented in the EMR, and another 35 percent said that they did not know about documentation of relaxation therapy in EMR. Of the MTFs that reported CPT codes available for relaxation therapy, only 6 percent report that every episode is documented using the CPT codes they reported; almost 30 percent said relaxation therapy was documented often; and 35 percent said that they did not know about the frequency of CPT code use for relaxation therapy.

Abbreviations

AHLTA	Armed Forces Health Longitudinal Technology Application
CAM	complementary and alternative medicine
CAPER	Comprehensive Ambulatory Provider Encounter Record
CCS	Clinical Classifications Software
CPT	Current Procedural Terminology
DCoE	Department of Defense Centers of Excellence for Psychological Health and Traumatic Brain Injury
DoD	Department of Defense
FTE	full-time equivalent
GS	General Schedule
ICD-9	International Classification of Diseases, Ninth Revision
IM	integrative medicine
MDD	major depressive disorder
MHS	military health system
MTF	military treatment facility
NCCAM	National Center for Complementary and Alternative Medicine
NCCIH	National Center for Complementary and Integrative Health
NCRMD	National Capital Region Medical Directorate
NIH	National Institutes of Health
POC	point of contact
PTSD	posttraumatic stress disorder

SIDR   Standard Inpatient Data Record

TBI   traumatic brain injury

TED-I   TRICARE Encounter Data—Institutional

TED-NI   TRICARE Encounter Data—Non-Institutional

USAMRMC   U.S. Army Medical Research and Materiel Command

VA   Department of Veterans Affairs

VHA   Veterans Health Administration

References

Barnes, P. M., B. Bloom, R. L. Nahin, *Complementary And Alternative Medicine Use Among Adults and Children: United States, 2007,* Hyattsville, Md.: National Center for Health Statistics, Centers for Disease Control and Prevention, 2008.

Chou, R., A. Qaseem, V. Snow, D. Casey, J. T. Cross, P. Shekelle, and D. K. Owens, "Diagnosis and Treatment of Low Back Pain: A Joint Clinical Practice Guideline From the American College of Physicians and the American Pain Society," *Annals of Internal Medicine,* Vol. 147, No. 7, 2007, pp. 478–491.

Clarke, T. C., L. I. Black, B. J. Stussman, P. M. Barnes, and R. L. Nahin, "Trends in the Use of Complementary Health Approaches Among Adults: United States, 2002–2012," *National Health Statistics Reports,* Vol. 79, 2015, pp. 1–16.

DoD—*See* U.S. Department of Defense.

Goertz, C., B. P. Marriott, M. D. Finch, R. M. Bray, T. V. Williams, L. L. Hourani, L. S. Hadden, H. L. Colleran, and W. B. Jonas, "Military Report More Complementary and Alternative Medicine Use than Civilians," *Journal of Alternative and Complementary Medicine,* Vol. 19, No. 6, 2013, pp. 509–517.

Healthcare Analysis & Information Group, *2011 Complementary and Alternative Medicine Survey,* Washington, D.C.: Department of Veterans Affairs, 2011.

Institute of Medicine Committee on the Use of Complementary and Alternative Medicine by the American Public, *Complementary and Alternative Medicine in the United States,* Washington, D.C.: National Academies Press, 2005.

Jacobson, I. G., M. R. White, T. C. Smith, B. Smith, T. S. Wells, G. D. Gackstetter, E. Boyko, and Millennium Cohort Study, "Self-Reported Health Symptoms and Conditions Among Complementary and Alternative Medicine Users in a Large Military Cohort," *Annals of Epidemiology,* Vol. 19, No. 9, 2009, pp. 613–622.

Kent, J. B., and R. C. Oh, "Complementary and Alternative Medicine Use Among Military Family Medicine Patients in Hawaii," *Military Medicine,* Vol. 175, No. 7, 2010, pp. 534–538.

Libby, D. J., C. E. Pilver, and R. Desai, "Complementary and Alternative Medicine in VA Specialized PTSD Treatment Programs, *Psychiatric Services,* Vol. 63, No. 11, 2012, pp. 1134–1136.

Lott, C. M., "Integration of Chiropractic in the Armed Forces Health Care System," *Military Medicine,* Vol. 161, No. 12, 1996, pp. 755–759.

Management of MDD Working Group, *VA/DoD Clinical Practice Guideline for Management of Major Depressive Disorder (MDD),* Washington, D.C.: Office of Quality and Performance, Department of Veterans Affairs, 2009.

Management of Post-Traumatic Stress Working Group, *VA/DoD Clinical Practice Guideline for Management of Post-Traumatic Stress,* Washington, D.C.: Department of Veteran Affairs, 2010. As of May 27, 2016: http://www.healthquality.va.gov/ptsd/ptsd-full-2010a.pdf

McPherson, L. F., and M. A. Schwenka, "Use of Complementary and Alternative Therapies Among Active Duty Soldiers, Military Retirees, and Family Members at a Military Hospital," *Military Medicine,* Vol. 169, No. 5, 2004, pp. 354–357.

Menard, M., A. Nielsen, H. Tick, W. Meeker, K. Wilson, and J. Weeks, "Never Only Opioids," in R. Payne, B. Twillman, S. A. Hussain, T. Galblum, and C. Leyland, eds., *Policy Brief*, Kansas City, Mo.: U.S. Cancer Pain Relief Fund, 2014.

National Center for Complementary Alternative Medicine, "What is Complementary and Alternative Medicine (CAM)?" web page, updated May 2012. As of August 1, 2016:
https://nccih.nih.gov/sites/nccam.nih.gov/files/D347_05-25-2012.pdf

National Center for Complementary and Integrative Health, "Complementary, Alternative, or Integrative Health: What's In a Name?" web page, National Institutes of Health, last updated March 2015a. As of May 27, 2016:
https://nccih.nih.gov/health/integrative-health

National Center for Complementary and Integrative Health, "Health Topics A–Z," web page, National Institutes of Health, last updated July 6, 2015b. As of May 27, 2016:
https://nccih.nih.gov/health/atoz.htm

NCCIH—*See* National Center for Complementary and Integrative Health.

Office of Personnel Management, "Salary Table 2015-GS, Incorporating the 1% General Schedule Increase, Effective January 2015," web page, 2015. As of May 26, 2016:
https://www.opm.gov/policy-data-oversight/pay-leave/salaries-wages/salary-tables/pdf/2015/GS.pdf

OPM—*See* Office of Personnel Management.

Petri Jr., R. P., and R. E. Delgado, "Integrative Medicine Experience in the U.S. Department of Defense," *Medical Acupuncture,* Vol. 27, No. 5, 2015, pp. 328–334.

Smith, T. C., M. A. Ryan, B. Smith, R. J. Reed, J. R. Riddle, G. R. Gumbs, and G. C. Gray, "Complementary and Alternative Medicine Use Among U.S. Navy and Marine Corps Personnel," *BMC Complementary and Alternative Medicine*, Vol. 7, No. 1, 2007, p. 16.

U.S. Department of Defense, *Integrative Medicine in the Military Health System Report to Congress,* Washington, D.C., 2014.

White, M. R., I. G. Jacobson, B. Smith, T. S. Wells, G. D. Gackstetter, E. J. Boyko, and T. C. Smith, "Health Care Utilization Among Complementary and Alternative Medicine Users in a Large Military Cohort," *BMC Complementary and Alternative Medicine*, Vol. 11, No. 1, 2011, p. 27.